# The N Guid to Managed Care

Susan Odegaard Turner, RN, MN, MBA, PhD
Chief Executive Officer
Turner Healthcare Associates, Inc.
Thousand Oaks, California

Project Staff
California Strategic Planning Committee for Nursing
Irvine, California

Assistant Clinical Professor
UCLA School of Nursing
Los Angeles, California

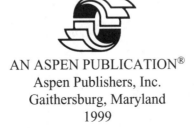

AN ASPEN PUBLICATION®
Aspen Publishers, Inc.
Gaithersburg, Maryland
1999

Library of Congress Cataloging-in-Publication Data

Turner, Susan Odegaard.
The nurse's guide to managed care/Susan Odegaard Turner.
p. cm.
Includes index.
ISBN 0-8342-1235-8
1. Nursing—Effect of managed care on. I. Title.
RT82 .T87 1999
362.1'73—ddc21
98-44092
CIP

Orders: (800) 638-8437
Customer Service: (800) 234-1660

**About Aspen Publishers** • For more than 35 years, Aspen has been a leading professional publisher in a variety of disciplines. Aspen's vast information resources are available in both print and electronic formats. We are committed to providing the highest quality information available in the most appropriate format for our customers. Visit Aspen's Internet site for more information resources, directories, articles, and a searchable version of Aspen's full catalog, including the most recent publications: **http://www.aspenpublishers.com**
**Aspen Publishers, Inc.** • The hallmark of quality in publishing
Member of the worldwide Wolters Kluwer group.

Editorial Services: Ruth Bloom
Library of Congress Catalog Card Number: 98-44092
ISBN: 0-8342-1235-8

*Printed in the United States of America*

1   2   3   4   5

# Dedication

This manuscript is dedicated to those who were my mentors in the beginning of my nursing career. Most of us can identify a few people who truly made a difference in our professional lives. Because of the things these individuals taught us, we made choices we might not have made otherwise. Fortunately, some of them are still available to mentor me!

I have a deep debt of gratitude to my mentors. Carol Ross Portnoy, Vicki Cashman Russell, Pat Odegaard, Patricia Cunningham, and the late Elizabeth Reece have all showed me what the best of the best in nursing is all about. Thank you for sharing with me. I salute you!

# Table of Contents

# Foreword

Consider this book your survival kit.

Health care is so vastly different than it was 10 years ago—and there's still so much change in the works—that every nurse, no matter what specialty, role, or level of education needs some guidance from time to time about how to best be successful, productive, and happy in the profession.

Experts predict that the nation's health care economy will grow to more than $300 billion by 2002 and will involve at least 15% of the gross domestic product. Mergers and acquisitions will continue to increase as a result of managed care. Health care companies recorded 1,183 merger or acquisition transactions in 1997, a 19% increase over the 997 deals reported in 1996 and an 87% rise over the 633 deals announced in 1995. Among hospitals, there were 181 mergers or acquisitions in 1997, up from 169 in 1996 and 133 in 1995.

For every one of these changes, scores of nurses are scrambling for good advice. In the wake of each merger and acquisition there is a wide range of new programs and procedures, some new jobs, some lost jobs, and much stress.

In order to thrive with all the new rules and roles, expectations and systems, nurses need a broad and solid understanding of why all these changes are occurring, and a clear road map to the future. Perhaps most importantly, nurses also must understand what specific skills they may need in the new millennium, and where their acumen can best be applied.

This book offers all that, and more. From insight on the history of the changes we are now witnessing to practical tips about new opportunities and necessary skills, *The Nurse's Guide to Managed Care* provides great guidance and information. There are concise summaries of the major issues facing the profession, but there also are specific ideas about how nurses can take action to better craft their careers to meet the demands managed care will continue to create.

As Susan Odegaard Turner points out, nursing *is* managed care, in the best sense of the word. Since the beginning of the century, expert nurses have been shepherding the care of acute and chronic patients in homes, clinics, and hospitals. Much has changed since those early days, but much has stayed the same. It's our job as nurses to develop a strong enough understanding of the needs of the system, of our own skills and strengths and those of our communities, that we can—collectively and individually—actively help craft the emerging system.

—*Barbara Bronson Gray, RN, MN*
Editor-in-Chief, *NurseWeek* and *HealthWeek*
Sunnyvale, California
Assistant Clinical Professor
UCLA School of Nursing
Los Angeles, California

# Introduction

## DEALING WITH THE FUTURE BY LOOKING TO THE PAST

In January 1998, Mary Grayson, editor of *Hospitals and Health Networks*, published an editorial (Grayson, 1998) that discussed some of the more difficult health care issues we are facing in the United States today. The irony of the editorial was that she used quotations from the early part of this century to describe our current dilemmas. Grayson came across old issues of American Hospital Association (AHA) newsletters from the 1920s and 1930s. Here are some of the issues Grayson found.

- The chaotic state of existing legislation relating to hospitals has been time and again pointed out, and to that end the association shall set up some machinery at headquarters to render much needed assistance to the field. *—William H. Walsh, MD, 1928*
- In 1928, the AHA printed a survey of "per-caput-diem costs." But it noted that hospitals reporting the data probably didn't use a standard cost accounting system, which would explain to some extent the wide difference in the costs of two hospitals in the same city. *—AHA, 1928*
- It must be fully recognized...that the care of the sick has expanded so as to include the care of the health of the entire community. *—John A. Hartwell, 1929*
- It is to be hoped...that all of us will have learned that to dismiss patients from the hospital just as soon as it may properly be done is an obligation which should not be ignored. *—Charles S. Woods, 1932*

Ms. Grayson noted that which all nurses must consider. The issues in health care are not new, nor can they be ignored. This book describes some of the issues and options affecting nurses in the new health care environment. Becoming more educated and informed about these issues allows all nurses to make an impact on the most important reason we all became nurses—the patients!

---

**BIBLIOGRAPHY**

Grayson, M. 1998. "Back to the Future!" *Hospitals and Health Networks*, 20 January, 7.

# CHAPTER 1

# Nursing: A Profession at the Crossroads

Nurses are being profoundly affected by the changes in the health care industry. These changes have caused complex issues and strong emotions to come to the forefront as the nursing profession struggles to find its place in the new health care marketplace.

Rapid changes occurring in health care due to marketplace reform and competition have had many effects. One of the most notable is the changing power base of players within the **health care system**. In most industries, the **consumer** makes the purchasing decision and pays for the product or service. In health care, the purchasing decision, payment, and receipt of services are separated (Teisberg et al., 1994). As a result, there are numerous tiers of customers: employers, who purchase health care coverage for their employees; third-party **payers**, such as insurance companies and health maintenance organizations, which collect premiums and then pay providers for services rendered to their subscribers; **patients**, who ultimately receive the health care services; and physicians, who determine or advise on tests and treatments for patients.

There are conflicting interests and priorities among these different customers. The employer wants to pay the lowest premiums. The third-party payer wants to pay less on patient care than it collects in premiums. The patient wants the best **quality of care** regardless of cost. The physician wants to correctly diagnose the patient but also be protected from litigation. These conflicting issues and interests have had dramatic impact on **hospitals** (Teisberg et al., 1994).

Because most of the 2.5 million nurses in this country (**ANA**, 1994) work in acute care hospitals, health care market readjustments have affected nurses significantly. One major consequence for nurses is the loss of thousands of acute care hospital jobs throughout the country as hospitals **downsize** and "rightsize" for the new marketplace. Hospitals have always been in the illness care business. With limited resources and competing customers, hospitals are evolving into a new arena of care—the newly integrated **health care delivery system** business.

The skill mix required for providing nursing care in this newly integrated system environment is different than the set of skills the registered nurse uses in the acute care setting. The requirements of the registered nurse role are changing as well. Many hospitals are replacing professional nurses with **unlicensed assistive personnel** (UAP) as caregivers. Even nurses with highly specialized training and extensive experience will be competing for jobs—especially those without advanced or baccalaureate degrees. **Differentiated nursing practice** based on education and competency is also increasing due to changes in health care delivery. Specific examples of dealing with these issues are discussed in later chapters.

**Integrated delivery systems** no longer allow the hospital to be the center of care and technology it once was (Lumsdon, 1994a). Earlier in this century, hospitals were places where people went when they were dying. Then came the technological revolution, and hospitals became centers of the latest technology and newest procedures. Hospitals are now expected to become large intensive care units, with only the costliest and most sophisticated care being provided there. The majority of care will be given out in the **community**, at a variety of sites with a multitude of different providers (Lumsdon, 1994a).

Many hospitals have assumed that reengineering and redesign of hospital clinical roles will allow nursing staff to successfully navigate the changes required for facilities to be successful in this new environment. After spending significant dollars on reengineering and redesign, some hospitals have discovered that nurses have not adapted to the new roles and functions at all—in fact, nurses have grown increasingly militant and hostile!

What's behind this new wave of resistance? Reengineering and redesign are not effective tools to change the way nurses view themselves and their profession. Reengineering and redesign do not deal with the emotional realities and human issues that the changing **nursing role** has invariably evoked. Missing from these organizational processes are the recognition of the intense **culture shock** nurses are experiencing and the means to assist them in dealing with transition.

Most hospitals have been designed with the "illness model" in mind. Patients come to the hospital for care during an acute episode of illness or to recover from surgery. The model of health care delivery that is evolving nationally is one based on wellness and prevention—the idea that patients receive care in the community—and de-emphasizes hospital admissions. This fundamental change in the health care delivery model poses a myriad of issues for the nursing profession, role, and function.

Hospitals have attempted to cope with these issues through reengineering and work redesign. The reengineering that has taken place in many hospitals has not changed systems or processes, but has simply changed the time frame within which nursing care is given. Nurses are being asked to provide the same level of care as always, but over a shorter time span.

One model of care that is now popular in acute care hospitals is that of patient-focused care (Bergman, 1994). This model of care involves bringing all the services to the patient in a decentralized way. The goal is to provide more continuity of care by having the patient interact with a minimum number of hospital staff.

Many patient care models did not create a new wellness model to accompany the newly integrated delivery system concepts outlined above, but simply compacted the hospitalization time. The nursing care pace has been significantly accelerated, which has caused frustration for many nursing staff.

The level of change now taking place for registered nurses is on a par with the changes overturning the aerospace, airline, and banking industries, to name just a few. But, in contrast to what has happened in other fields—where difficult decisions are being faced squarely and tough programs are being implemented to adapt organizations to new realities—nursing has not been able to make the necessary changes successfully.

## THE CHANGING NATURE OF NURSING

Nursing came into being as a response to human needs, to the needs of all persons for security, comfort, care, and support during varying states of health (Harrington and Estes, 1997). Because of this beginning, nursing has been and will continue to be part of the basic fabric of society. Nursing traditionally has been a female profession and has included tasks such as bathing, feeding, and changing soiled linens. These basic personal care tasks have often caused nurses to be looked at as handmaidens and menial laborers by physicians and other health care team members.

V.A. Lanara describes the core of nursing as care and service (1993). She states that care runs through nursing literature as a theme from Greek classical writings to the Florence Nightingale period. Caring for and about patients is a unifying force in nursing, according to Dr. Lanara. It frames a compelling picture of persistence in the face of internal and external pressureto promote the case for the direct care every patient needs. Once again, nursing is facing pressure to provide care.

According to Virginia Henderson, in 1978, another basic element of nursing is service (Harrington and Estes, 1997). It is considered a universal aspect of nursing that is intimate, constant, and comforting. Care and service are nursing's historical and ideological foundations, and are perpetuated by nurses in the 1990s.

Nurses now also have additional roles besides bedside care and service. They are expected to act as "family nurses" who know their individual patients' health needs and collaborate with other members of the health team for effective coverage of those needs (Harrington and Estes, 1997). Nurses are also expected to be social missionaries for health and to participate in society's efforts to fight social evils such as child endangerment as well as health-damaging behaviors such as chemical addiction and smoking. In addition to these new roles, nurses must now prove that their services are unique, of high value, cost-effective, and absolutely necessary in today's evolving health care environment.

It is difficult to articulate all of the changes occurring in the nursing profession. All of us within nursing can feel the differences, and share the grief and pain caused by the recognition that nursing as many of us have known it is no longer viable. Twenty years ago, nurses could choose between employers, work a variety of schedules, and determine the perks to accompany a job that was virtually guaranteed for life as long as one stayed clinically competent. The changes in employment conditions since then have been dramatic. In 1996, for instance, 200 nurses applied for six new graduate internship spots in a local hospital, and other facilities throughout the country downsized registered nurse positions in waves. By 1998, California began to experience a **nursing shortage** of skilled critical-care nurses (Gray, 1994a). For nurses and nursing students, this roller coaster ride of raised employment expectations and dashed hopes is incredibly frightening.

The "unchanging rules" that nurses have been familiar with in nursing seem to be no longer valid or in force. Clinical competence as a guarantee of employment, eternal job security, and all-RN staffing models are concepts of the past, and their disappearance has caused culture shock for many experienced nurses working in hospitals. As more and more hospitals reengineer and redesign, nurses become overwhelmed, hostile, defensive, antagonistic, and militant. **Union** activity is becoming increasingly common in traditionally nonunion facilities. Transition into a new way of thinking and practicing nursing has not been evident nor welcomed by nurses in many hospitals.

To understand the evolution that is taking place within nursing, and to assess future directions for the profession, it is helpful to evaluate past behaviors. The medical practice model created the role of nurses as handmaidens to physicians; not as collaborative colleagues, but as subordinates. This role was accepted by the nursing profession, which, like other traditionally female professions, took its subservient status for granted.

Nursing has often allowed other disciplines to dictate its practice and role direction—and given away pieces of itself in the process. For instance, respiratory therapists, physical therapists, and occupational therapists determined that they would be responsible for portions of care previously administered by nurses, and nursing gave away those components, believing that to do so would add, not subtract, from its patient advocacy power base.

These changes seemed minuscule and unimportant at the time they took place, and in fact were welcomed as ways to give nurses more time to do nursing. But as a result, many non-nurse hospital administrators and others without a clinical mindset do not understand exactly what nurses do and why nurses are valuable. Patient care reengineering and redesign efforts therefore have failed to recognize and deal with the culture shift and role changes nurses must make to be successful.

The changes within the profession of nursing might be compared to changes to the structure of a building. The foundation of the profession remains the same. The cornerstones of the profession are shifting. The foundation has always been patient advocacy and maximum beneficial outcomes. The cornerstones have been meeting patient needs and providing the best care without regard to cost. The pillars have been specialization with narrow focus, and no expectation of flexibility. The pillars are now under renovation, changing to include minimal flexibility, an "us versus them" mentality, and professional in-fighting.

The foundation of the new nursing role remains the same, but what is needed now are new cornerstones—**primary care** generalists, integrated care, and community-wide focus. New pillars are needed also to ensure less duplication, flexibility, cross-training, and one unified professional voice.

Creating new roles requires nurses to adjust to a huge culture shift within nursing, and to deal with emotional realities. Role definitions, specific tasks, and interrelated functions must be created for registered nurses, **licensed vocational nurses**, and unlicensed assistive personnel. Nurses must define their role in the new health care delivery business, and clarify to non-nurse providers and players why that role is cost-effective, innovative, and unique in its functions. Expanded nursing roles will be addressed in Chapter 17. Core **competencies** of the nurses for the future are discussed in Chapters 14 and 17.

Because this role adjustment is so difficult and frightening to many, some nurses have become defensive, mistrusting, or militant. There is both risk and potential if physicians, non-clinical administrators, and labor organizations begin to define the nursing role and **nursing practice** because nursing has not yet done so in a unified way. Nurses are being called on to reinvent a unique and expansive new role for themselves on their own in this new health care arena. Allowing nursing labor unions to create this redefinition of nurses may foster a focus only concerned with collective bargaining issues and minimize the potential that now exists to enhance nursing roles. Discussion of nursing labor and **collective bargaining** organizations will take place in Chapter 16.

## TRANSITION STRATEGIES

It is clear that hospitals and other health care providers must continue to change the way they provide care. However, reengineering and redesign methods that do not incorporate nursing culture changes, transition management, and professional nursing issues and solutions are doomed to failure, as many organizations have discovered.

The primary cause of nurses' hostility during organizational transition may be the inability to understand that change is mandatory for hospitals' survival. Unfortunately, many nurses have been unable to participate proactively in creating the changes nurses are expected to make. Without bricks, there are no walls, and many nurses are having a difficult time redesigning new bricks.

It is time to create a new future. Clearly defining new expectations and expanding existing parameters can be difficult for those nurses who have never had a unified voice or been personally accountable for their professional direction. Many nurses have focused effectively on patient advocacy, without focusing on the system. Pioneering nursing professionals are starting to break out of the old ways of thinking and are beginning to change nursing's professional framework.

It will take years to move nursing through the present professional identity crisis. In the meantime, nurses must be assisted through the quagmire of ongoing patient care changes. Tools are needed for nurses to progress to the next stage. Nurses also need education and communication from administrators and nurse executives to change the future of nursing.

Some nurses are already out there trying to find the answers. They are looking at redefining undergraduate curricula, building advanced nursing practice programs, and designing **managed care** training programs. There are **nursing transitions skills** imparted through health care programs provided by professional nurse specialty groups. Certification programs for quality improvement, health care leadership, and other subjects also are available. One organization, American Association of Critical-Care Nurses (AACN), based in Aliso Viejo, California, is helping its members cope with change by offering a five-part training program entitled, "Transitions in Healthcare." Other specialty organizations have developed training programs to assist registered nurses with professional transition. Some even offer a transition kit for members.

Nurse innovators all across the country are leading the organizational changes in their hospitals, systems, and emerging integrated delivery **networks** by implementing unique and creative patient care options that decrease lengths of stay, lower costs, and enhance patient outcomes. The case studies used throughout this book outline successful examples of innovative and effective changes in health care delivery that enhance the nursing role and practice.

These nurses are looking outside traditional nursing boundaries and leading the charge toward building clinical pathways, developing multidisciplinary teams, and coordinating efforts among doctors, nurses, and other allied health care professionals to respond to the demands of managed care and systems integration. Successful models of patient care delivery in a multitude of settings and organization-building for the new era will emerge more clearly.

Readers who are not nurses will be stymied by some of the professional issues nurses struggle with. Non-clinical administrators will wonder why some of these issues need to be addressed at all and will be at a loss for innovative ways to deal with the changing nursing culture. Others will wonder how to undo the changes in their facilities that have caused their nurses so much turmoil.

The core strategies for moving forward are really quite simple: educate and communicate with nurses. Some innovative ideas are outlined in this book. Others will be developed in hospitals across the country. Frank discussions of many of the current nursing issues outlined here will allow non-nurses to see inside the nursing culture and understand what values underpin the nursing role and provision of nursing care. The case studies and expanded role examples can assist with reflection on and assessment of nursing care provision options.

These are exciting times for the nursing profession. Nurses can now focus energy on managing the transition into a new health care arena. Nurses can be helped to recognize and embrace the changes that are needed. Above all, the unique, valuable, and essential role that nurses provide in health care today will be clearly identified and understood by those outside the nursing profession.

## DISCUSSION QUESTIONS

1. How has the practice of nursing changed in your geographic area? Why?
2. What are the five most pressing issues for nursing in your geographic area? Why?
3. What are the five most pressing issues for health care consumers in your geographic area?
4. Are the answers to questions 2 and 3 related? Why or why not?

---

**BIBLIOGRAPHY**

American Nurses' Association. 1985. *Code for Nurses*. Washington, D.C.: ANA Publishing.

————. 1993. *Nursing's Agenda for Health Care Reform*. Washington, D.C.: ANA Publishing.

————. 1994. *Every Patient Deserves a Nurse*. Brochure. Washington, D.C.: ANA Publishing.

————. 1995. *Nursing's Social Policy Statement*. Washington, D.C.: ANA Publishing.

————. 1996. *Scope and Standards of Advanced Practice Registered Nursing*. Washington, D.C.: ANA Publishing.

Bergman, R. 1994. "Reengineering Health Care." *Hospitals and Health Networks*, 5 February, 16–24.

Beyers, M. 1996. "The Value of Nursing." *Hospitals and Health Networks*, 5 February, 6.

Curran, C., ed. 1990. "IDN Core Competencies and Nursing's Role." *Nursing Economics*, December, 1.

Dillon, P. 1997. "The Future of Associate Degree Nursing." *Nursing and Healthcare: Perspectives on Community*, January/February, 12–15.

Donaho, B., ed. 1996. *Celebrating the Journey: A Final Report on Strengthening Hospital Nursing*. Philadelphia: National Academy Press.

Goldsmith, J. 1993. "Driving the Nitroglycerin Truck." *Healthcare Forum Journal*, March/April, 36–44.

————. 1996. "Managed Care Mythology: Supply Dreams Die Hard." *Healthcare Forum Journal*, November/December, 43–47.

Gray, B.B. 1994a. "Twenty-First Century Hospital Embodies New Concept." *NurseWeek*, 1 April, 1.

————. 1994b. "Changing Skill Mix Reorders Healthcare Delivery System." *NurseWeek*, 2 December, 14.

————. 1995a. "Nurses Face Ethics of Rationing as Healthcare Industry Evolves." *NurseWeek*, 2 April, 20–22.

————. 1995b. "Issues at the Crossroads." Parts 1 and 2. *NurseWeek*, 1 October, 1.

Grayson, M. 1998. "Back to the Future." *Hospitals and Health Networks*, 20 January, 7.

Hall, G. et al. 1993. "How to Make Reengineering Really Work." *Harvard Business Review*, November/December, 119–131.

Harrington, C., and Estes, C., eds. 1997. *Health Policy and Nursing*. 2nd ed. Boston: Jones and Bartlett.

Koerner, J.G., and Karpiuk, K.L. 1994. *Implementing Differentiated Nursing Practice: Transformation by Design*. Gaithersburg, MD: Aspen Publishers, Inc.

Lanara, V.A. 1993. "The Nurse of the Future, Role and Function." *Journal of Nursing Management* 1: 83–87.

Lumsdon, K. 1994a. "It's a Jungle Out There!" *Hospitals and Health Networks*, 20 May, 68–72.

————. 1994b. "Want to Save Millions?" *Hospitals and Health Networks*, 5 November, 24–32.

————. 1995. "Working Smarter, Not Harder." *Hospitals and Health Networks*, 5 November, 27–31.

Organization of Nurse Leaders. 1995. Focus Group Notes. *Nursing Issues*. 29 September.

Pew Health Professions Commission. 1995. "Healthy America: Practitioners for 2005." *Pew Health Professions Report*. Washington, D.C.: Pew Health Professions Commission.

————. 1998. *Pew Health Professions Report*. Pew Health Professions Commission.

Sherer, J. 1994. "Job Shifts." *Hospitals and Health Networks*, 5 October, 64–68.

Shubert, D. 1996. "Hospitals Decrease Nurses' Role: Reassign Tasks to Aides." *Los Angeles Times*, 14 July, 1.

Teisberg, E. et al. 1994. "Making Competition in Health Care Work." *Harvard Business Review*, July/August, 131–141.

Turner, S.O. 1995a. "Managing Your Transition: Strategies for the Future." *Surgical Services Management*, May, 40–42.

————. 1995b. "Reality Check: It's Time for Nursing to Face the Future." *Hospitals and Health Networks*, 20 August, 20–22.

————. 1996. "Capitation: Are You Ready for It?" *Surgical Services Management*, February, 43–45.

# CHAPTER 2

# Nursing and Managed Care: A Reality Check

Change is sweeping across the health care industry, uprooting people, institutions, and professions in rapid succession. The nursing profession is no exception; indeed, even as nurses continue to react with shock and dismay to changes careening their way, the pace of transformation in their field is actually quickening.

At a fundamental level, nursing is being forced to reinvent itself. Faced with escalating costs and the need to integrate the fragmented pieces of the delivery system into coherent new wholes, hospital and other health care executives are rewriting nurses' roles through initiatives with names like reengineering, patient-centered care, critical paths and outcomes management.

Finding themselves consistently near the eye of the storm, hospital-based nurses are working harder than ever before to provide quality patient care. But given the fundamental shifts taking place all around them, no health care professionals have been as surprised and unprepared for the massive change in their field.

The level of change now taking place for nurses is on a par with the changes overturning the aerospace, airline, and banking industries, to

*Source:* Reprinted from *Hospitals and Health Networks,* Vol. 69, No. 16, by permission August 20, 1995, Copyright 1995, American Hospital Publishing, Inc.

name a few. But in contrast to what's happened in other fields, where difficult decisions are being faced squarely and tough programs are being implemented to move organizations to where they need to be, many nurses are fighting change every step of the way. What's behind this wave of nurse resistance?

No one is pretending that the changes in health care aren't being dictated in large part by the mushrooming cost of the system. Nurses oppose many of the current redesign efforts because they believe care quality is being compromised, and that the new systems being put into place are ineffective. We haven't successfully managed the transition into a new way of thinking; the implementation of patient-centered care and the restructuring of hospital-based organizations have left nurses more hostile and defiant than ever.

The biggest problem is the inability of many nurses to deal with transition and change—to accept that change is mandatory for organizational survival. One reason for this is the fact that many hospital administrators without a clinical mindset have created a kind of Catch-22 for their nursing staffs. Under the guise of "cost-saving initiatives," hospitals have eliminated support positions for nursing while simultaneously laying off thousands of nurses, especially RNs. This kind of short-term thinking has resulted in nurses taking on other ancillary roles.

This is an expensive way to adapt to change and extremely frustrating for nurses, who are already doing more for sicker patients over shorter lengths of stay. The result? Nursing staff morale has plummeted, while professional frustration, victimization and union activism have increased.

Because many nurses are frightened, angry, and confused, some are turning to organized nursing groups, believing that those groups will provide them with magic answers and painless solutions.

Not surprisingly, large groups like the American Nurses' Association have taken aggressive public stances in an effort to bolster their membership rolls. Commentaries and marketing materials from the association and other organizations tend to convey the message that all nurses should oppose the evolution the delivery system is going through.

In fact, there are nurses in this country who support the changes taking place. Many of those individuals recognize the potential that systemic change holds for nurses, a potential that could at last bring nurses to the strategic decision-making table in ways not even dreamed of 20 years ago.

These nurses believe that the nursing role should be expanded and enhanced; that delegation of nonprofessional tasks to trained, unlicensed caregivers closely supervised by RNs doesn't automatically lower care quality; and that opposing change for the sake of doing so is demeaning and obstructive.

It's important to remember that the ANA and its local chapters represent only about 10 percent of all nurses in this country. Organized nursing simply is not a major voice for the nursing profession. To add to the confusion, organized nursing groups have led the general public to believe that the issues are declining care quality matched by poor clinical outcomes, the logical results (in their view) of the restructuring and downsizing of hospitals, the changes taking place in the RN staffing mix, and hospitals' plans to maximize profits at the expense of quality.

The irony here is that nurses have left those without a clinical mindset to make the decisions about patient care, because they've been too busy fighting to proactively participate.

Meanwhile, the public's response to the soapbox oratory coming from organized nursing is confusion and misunderstanding. Most health care consumers would agree that they want RNs rather than unlicensed personnel to care for them, but last November's election—and a slew of opinion polls—also confirm that they don't want to pay more for anything. Amid conflicting reports and research on staffing levels and skill-mix patterns in hospitals, most members of the public are collectively throwing up their hands and demanding that we "change the system—just don't ask me to pay for it!"

At the same time, ANA activities that fight creative approaches to staffing, restructuring and work redesign leave many nurses believing that needed changes can be prevented if they fight hard enough and resist them long enough.

The tough reality is that these aren't the issues at all. The ANA is asking the wrong questions and overlooking the right answers. The real issues are not about staffing, cutting **FTEs** (Full Time Equivalents), or patient outcomes; they're about changing the culture of nursing and the nursing role, about fear and powerlessness, about lack of control and lack of input into the process. Nurses' fear and anger are really about fear of the unknown, fear that what has always worked won't work anymore, anger that the culture that nursing has created for itself has led to narrow focus, specialization, and fragmentation—approaches that don't work anymore.

Let's face facts: Nurses no longer control the marketplace, their salaries, or perks. And while issues like entry into practice, speaking as a unified professional voice, and lack of broad, agreed-on goals are talked about constantly within the profession, the reality never changes. Nurses need to stop bickering over definitions and begin changing the boundaries of the paradigm. Unfortunately, many nurses aren't yet ready to accept the changes that are required in a refocused health care environment. Some individuals haven't had the benefit of the education and communication needed to prepare for the future. Others are so frustrated by hospitals' "ready-fire-aim" cost-cutting initiatives that they've become militant. The ANA could help nurses through the transition process, but it's chosen instead to maintain nurses' sense of victimization in the face of change.

It is tempting to assume that this historic sentiment is primarily a throwback to nursing's status as a traditionally female profession and to nurses' old conditioning as handmaidens of doctors. While this may be part of the problem, a lack of conflict resolution skills and a persistent tendency to behave like codependent victims are also driving much of nursing's current mentality.

It's time to leave that mindset behind. How many hospital CEOs do you see picketing in the streets? Health care executives are out there trying to shift their own paradigms, aware that the managed care revolution is forcing action on many levels. They may be making mistakes, but they're making decisions, and accepting the consequences of their actions.

Clearly defining new expectations and expanding existing parameters is a frightening process for those nurses who've never had a unified voice or been personally accountable for their profession. Many nurses have focused advocacy on the patients they care for, without focusing on the professional limitations of the system. Pioneering nursing professionals are starting to break out of the old ways of thinking and are beginning to do something about it.

They are also recognizing a fundamental fact: The answers for nursing don't lie in the legislative process, in press conferences, in media marketing blitzes, or in marches on Washington. The answers will lie in accountability, proactive transitioning work, and the search for new options.

Nurses needs tools to progress to the next stage. What we need to be talking about is not how things have always been, but instead what the possibilities and strategies will be for the twenty-first century.

And some nurses are out there trying to find the answers. They're looking at redefining undergraduate curricula, building advanced nursing practice programs and designing managed care training programs. Nurse innovators all across the country are leading the organizational changes in their hospitals, systems, and emerging integrated delivery networks by implementing unique and creative patient care options that decrease lengths of stay, lower costs, and enhance patient outcomes.

These nurses are leading the charge toward building clinical pathways, developing multidisciplinary care teams and coordinating efforts among doctors, nurses, and other allied health care professionals to respond to the demands of managed care and systems integration.

One group assisting nurse leaders in the process is the American Organization of Nurse Executives. Another group, the American Association of Critical-Care Nurses, is designing transition training to assist critical care nurses in the new marketplace. As these and other organizations work to find solutions, successful models of patient care delivery and organization-building for the new era will emerge more clearly.

This is an arena with so much potential for nursing. The organized nursing groups now capitalizing on the current anxiety could join the transitioning process instead of encouraging their members to fear and resist change.

Nurses can take heart in knowing that they will be a vital component in the new integrated delivery systems. Indeed, with higher patient acuity and the need to build a real continuum of care across many sites, there's no question the challenges facing us will be insurmountable without the input and participation of nursing professionals. The core strategies for moving forward are really quite simple: educate and communicate. Nurses need to help one another through the tremendous process of change facing both their profession and the health care delivery system.

I am proud to be a nurse; while I no longer give bedside care, my nursing soul affects the work I do every day. These are exciting times for my profession. It's time for all of us to focus our energies on managing the transition for nurses and for our organizations, and on helping nurses to recognize and embrace the changes that are needed.

It's time to push past feelings of job entitlement and rigidity, and encourage one another to see that it's up to each of us to help create a new culture in health care. It's time to recognize and exercise the power each one of us has to participate in the shaping of the new delivery system to the benefit of our patients.

## DISCUSSION QUESTIONS

1. What behaviors, emotions, attitudes, and characteristics do you see in nurses involved in managed care? Why?
2. What is nursing's most important role in managed care? What are the causes for these?
3. How should nurses best be utilized in a managed care-based health care delivery system? Why?
4. Give three examples of nursing advocacy for patients.

---

**BIBLIOGRAPHY**

American Nurses' Association. 1993. *Nursing's Agenda for Health Care Reform*. Washington, D.C.: ANA Publishing.

————. 1994. *Every Patient Deserves a Nurse*. Brochure. Washington, D.C.: ANA Publishing.

————. 1996. *Registered Professional Nurses and Unlicensed Assistive Personnel*. 2nd ed. Washington, D.C.: ANA Publishing.

American Organization of Nurse Executives. 1996. *Talking Points on Hospital Redesign*. Washington, D.C.: American Organization of Nurse Executives.

Burda, D. 1994. "A Profit by Any Other Name Would Still Give Hospitals the Fits." *Modern Healthcare*, 8 August, 115–136.

————. 1995. "ANA Report Stokes Restructuring Debate." *Modern Healthcare*, 13 February, 38.

Burns, J. 1993. "Caring for the Community." *Modern Healthcare*, 8 November, 30–33.

California Nurses Association. Web Site Home Page. http://www.califnurses.org/

Coile, R. 1993a. "California Healthcare 2001: The Outlook for America's Bellwether State." *Hospital Strategy Report* 5(4), February, 1–3.

————. 1993b. "California Hospitals in the 21st Century." *California Hospitals*, November/December, 7–10.

————. 1994a. "Primary Care Networks: The Integrators of Care in an Integrated Delivery System." *Hospital Strategy Report* 6(8): 1–3.

————. 1994b. "Capitation: The New Food Chain of HMO Provider Payment." *Hospital Strategy Report* 6(9): 1–3.

Flower, J. 1997. "The Age of Heretics." *Healthcare Forum Journal*, March/April, 34–39.

Goldsmith, J. 1993. "Driving the Nitroglycerin Truck." *Healthcare Forum Journal*, March/April, 36–44.

———. 1996. "Managed Care Mythology: Supply Dreams Die Hard." *Healthcare Forum Journal*, November/December, 43–47.

Golub, E. 1995. "Revisiting Our Ideas about Health." *Hospitals and Health Networks*, 20 January, 78.

Goodman, J. 1993. *Twenty Myths about National Health Insurance*. National Center for Policy Analysis, Dallas, Texas.

Marks, M. 1994. *From Turmoil to Triumph*. New York: Lexington Press.

Pew Health Professions Commission. 1995. "Healthy America: Practitioners for 2005." *Pew Health Professions Report*. Washington, D.C.: Pew Health Professions Commission.

Turner, S.O. 1995a. "Marketing Yourself in the Nineties." *American Journal of Nursing*, January, 20–23.

———. 1995b. "Stand Out or Lose Out." *Nursing 95*, January, 13–18.

———. 1995c. "Laid Off: Now What?" *Nursing 95*, May, 94–95.

———. 1995d. "Managing Your Transition: Strategies for the Future." *Surgical Services Management*, May, 40–42.

———. 1995e. "Reality Check: It's Time for Nursing to Face the Future." *Hospitals and Health Networks*, 20 August, 20–22.

Udvarhelyi, I.S. et al. 1994. "Perspectives: Finding a Lasting Cure for US Healthcare." *Harvard Business Review*, September/October, 45–63.

Ummel, S. 1997. "Integration." *Healthcare Forum Journal*, March/April, 13–27.

Weissenstein, E., and Pallarito, K. 1994. "Senate Plan Adds to Reform Confusion." *Modern Healthcare*, 8 August, 2–4.

Wesorick, B. "Standards: On the Cutting Edge or Over the Cliff?" *Notes on Clinical Practice, 1990s*. Unpublished paper.

# CHAPTER 3

# The Evolving Health Care System

The traditional health care system that most nurses trained and worked in had standard and predictable characteristics. Today, as many experts have said, the only constant in health care is change.

## THE TRADITIONAL HEALTH CARE SYSTEM

In the traditional health care system, physicians were always in control of patients. They determined who needed hospital care and what type of care and treatment would be provided. They recommended the hospital the patient stayed in and the length of stay for each patient. Physicians practiced at one or two local community hospitals and rarely saw patients in other facilities. Hospital care was controlled and delivered by physician specialists in cardiology, surgery, respiratory, genitourinary, neurosurgery, and other specialties. Physician specialists were the power brokers in the hospital, and care provided outside the hospital was minimal.

Hospitals were seen as the major provider of care, and the center for technology. Patients chose their doctors and doctors chose the hospital in which to care for patients. High-technology equipment and procedures were provided by hospitals, and there was stiff competition to purchase the latest innovation in equipment.

Patients' care in hospitals was provided by health care personnel based on the hospital's individual determination of quality and satisfactory care. There were no staffing or acuity criteria. What seemed "right" for the patients was implemented. Measuring patient satisfaction and care quality was not a priority. Measurement of quality indicators has occurred only in the past 10 to 15 years. Hospital services and rituals were designed for hospital and provider convenience, not patient or payer. The focus of the patient care system was on illness and acute treatment. Patients sought care at the local hospital in their community regardless of cost or skills of providers at the facilities. Patients did not question the need for or costs of care regardless of probable outcomes or resources used. Health care was perceived as a right for all residents, even non-citizens, undocumented immigrants, and those without ability to pay for the care provided.

Previously, funds were controlled by providers—hospitals and physicians and were paid regardless of patient insurance status or cost of care. Physicians and hospitals were unconcerned about the cost of care; whatever the patient needed in order to be cared for was deemed appropriate and quality care. Paying for health care was not a concern. In 1965, the **Medicare** program was started, and provided unlimited entitlements from federal monies for health care of older Americans.

Additional federal funds such as Social Security and **Medicaid**, as well as state funds such as Aid to Families with Dependent Children, provided financial support for those with long-term disabilities or inability to pay for health care services. In the past, support has been unlimited to recipients of any of these funds, regardless of time on program, severity of need, or ability to work.

Medicare beneficiaries in 1997 totaled 38 million Americans, with an average outlay per beneficiary of $4,964 per year. The sickest 10 percent of the population average costs of $36,960 per year. Medicare's biggest outlay for a medical treatment is $5 billion a year for coronary bypass surgery. It is anticipated that Medicare beneficiaries in 2017 will equal 56 million, almost double the 1997 Medicare population. Lifetime Medicare taxes and premium payments for a man turning 65 in 1995 are estimated to be $35,000. His lifetime benefits used are close to $75,000. Lifetime Medicare taxes and premium payments for a woman turning 65 in 1995 are $46,000, with lifetime benefits used estimated at $111,000 (all sources: HCFA). As costs rise, it may be that the provision of health care is becoming a privilege for the insured, not a right for all Americans.

## THE EMERGING HEALTH CARE SYSTEM

The American health care system is constantly changing and evolving. Managed care is now the predominant method of caring for consumers, with **cost containment** strategies prioritized equally with quality. The number of Americans in managed health care plans in 1992 was 93 million. In 1996, it was 160 million (HCFA). The share of household income spent in 1996 for health care by households with members under 65 years of age was 3.7 percent; for those with members 65 and older it was 11.9 percent (HCFA). In both health care and political circles, there is debate as to whether the United States can afford a health care system that includes and provides care for over 40 million (1996 estimate) uninsured people.

The hospital is now seen as only one of many care providers in an integrated health care system and as part of the health care continuum. An integrated delivery system network is expected to deliver all needed care in a geographic region or marketplace. The focus of the evolving system is on wellness and prevention. Focus of the integrated health care system is on keeping patients out of high-cost environments (mainly hospitals) and providing care in **alternative delivery sites** whenever possible.

In this new delivery system, satisfaction of patients and payers is deemed critical and is necessary in order to continue successful contracting and patient relationship management. Educated consumers will shop for health care on the basis of price, service, access, and quality. All providers are expected to document and measure clinical outcomes, as well as adhere to clinical care guidelines, or critical pathways for patient **care management**. Communities demand total continuum of care and unlimited access.

Monetary funds and the integrated system are controlled by the biggest payers—employers and insurance companies—and require knowledgeable providers who know each payer system and individual contract provisions. Many payers and contract arrangements differ as to the information they request of providers when care is provided to members. Federal and state governments are capping (enforcing a maximum funding ceiling on) entitlements and restricting access by limiting qualified recipients. There is increased pressure from private sector business to limit costs of insurance premiums (employers won't pay more for employee coverage).

Marketplace competition is also forcing major reforms, such as revamping of federal and state entitlement programs like Medicare, including limitations on participants, and requiring higher out-of-pocket **deductibles** for enrollees. Ironically, according to some, Medicaid reimbursement is now higher than most managed care company reimbursement, while in the past it was at least 40 percent lower.

Hospitals are no longer just providing acute care—they are in the health care delivery system business. That is not the same business as the illness care business that hospitals were built to support, which means a new business imperative must be created in order for hospitals to be successful. Hospitals must manage costs and maintain quality as part of this health care delivery business. Hospitals, as well as physicians, are now expected to assume some of the financial risk of providing care. Hospitals must treat more complex patients using state-of-the-art technology, identifying anticipated clinical outcomes, and discharging the patients quickly. Patients must be educated to continue their care following discharge because they are now discharged much sooner. Patients must be educated to use **primary care physicians (PCPs)** first (even before coming to the emergency department, in some cases), and focus their health care priorities on wellness, screening, and prevention.

Hospitals and physicians are becoming partners in providing care. In fact, joint ventures between physicians and hospitals are commonplace in this new health care environment. **Management services organizations** (MSOs), **independent practice associations** (IPAs), and other arrangements bring hospitals and physicians together to contract with payers to provide health care services. Physicians in solo practice are increasingly rare. Physicians are partnering with each other as well, to form groups for contracting and providing services.

Health care is now driven by primary care and prevention, with primary care physicians as **gatekeepers** and specialists referred to only as needed in order to minimize cost. There is an ever-increasing need for primary care physicians and an excess of specialists caused by the changing health care expectations. To cope with the excess of providers, some payers create and maintain physician profiles that reflect the physician's practice pattern, length of stay, readmission rate, medical cost of care, and patient satisfaction. Based on physician profiles, contracts are negotiated with the most cost-effective quality care providers and patients are specifically directed to those physicians.

Medical care is also provided by caregivers in alternative sites like home health care, infusion centers, clinics, and schools by employing available technology such as car phones, laptop computers, telemanagement, and other strategies. Two **health maintenance organizations** (HMOs), Blue Shield of California and Health Net, have joined the growing ranks of medical groups offering **alternative treatment plans**. Beginning in January 1998, employers can purchase acupuncture riders to their health plans from both groups. Blue Shield also will launch a network of chiropractors, acupuncture practitioners, massage therapists, and stress management seminars, as well as discounts at fitness clubs and services. Health Net also includes chiropractor benefits (LA Times).

In a recent Harvard University Medical School study, more than one-third of respondents said they used at least one "unconventional therapy" during the past year (LA Times). Many physicians already use complementary and alternative therapies that they deem safe and effective.

Hospitals now must ensure good outcomes for patients and show that patients improve over time in order to prevent re-admissions and relapses, which force chronically ill patients to be managed outside the hospital on an ongoing basis and with alternative therapies. In addition, legislation has had to be created to deal with provider roles, functions, and turf battles between providers (such as between physicians and nurse practitioners, between emergency nurses and emergency medical technicians, and between physicians and midwives) because of efforts to lower costs and restructure the health care system.

## WHAT CAUSED THE CHANGES IN THE US HEALTH CARE SYSTEM?

Medical care costs were increasing faster than the gross national product in the 1980s. There were questions by health care analysts about whether the expense provided equivalent benefit. Information already existed about some forms of **capitated care** delivery, such as health maintenance organizations. There were also other studies that determined that public health measures, lifestyle choices, and social/environmental conditions related more to aggregate health than did use of medical services.

Others believed the use of regulation to control medical costs was needed because market forces in medical care could have only a marginal impact on medical spending. This ineffectiveness was due to the existence of extensive insurance coverage, which made patients uninterested in and unresponsive to the costs of insurance and medical education. Patient unresponsiveness in turn created an increased demand as well as supply of medical services.

Adding to the dilemma was the fact that patients do not behave like typical consumers when consuming medical services. They depend on physicians to make crucial and life-determining choices. Physicians and nurses, based on their training as patient advocates, tend to do as much as possible for their patients.

For whatever reason, in the 1980s large buyers of medical services, primarily insurance companies, did not have the power or did not use their power to require hospitals, physicians, and other health professionals to limit costs. Because of this lack of significant checks, the growth in medical services and expenses was extraordinary. As a result, incentives, markets, competition, and limited use of government regulation have slowed the rise in medical expenses. These changes have been significant, and to a large degree have increased efficiency.

Government regulation and competitive markets are different ways to allocate medical services, control costs, maintain quality, and choose public and social priorities. However, because of the unique nature of medical services and the medical sector, neither of these methods has been effective. There seems to be no political or social will to embrace either a competitive market system or a governmental regulatory approach. Some geographic regions of the country have experienced increased governmental involvement and regulation of health care as a method to deter motives considered not in the consumer's best interest. For example, California recently developed a legislative mandate that patients can receive reimbursement for emergency care rendered by a medical provider that a "reasonable and prudent person" would consider appropriate medical care for that complaint. This legislation grew out of the increasing discontent of health care consumers with payer denials of care when the patient considered the situation an emergency, but the payer, after the fact, did not.

What is lacking in the medical market are two of the most sought-after components of markets—competition that reduces price and budget constraints that control spending. Regulations that raise minimum standards of care contribute to the lack of price competitiveness. In addition, many people believe that medical care is a special service that should be allocated based on need. This prompts patients to demand extra precautions in diagnosis and treatment. The physician advocacy role also encourages this mindset. Therefore, there is rarely a reduced demand for medical services when prices rise, nor do providers lower prices significantly when faced with increased competition.

## THE INDUSTRY OF HEALTH CARE

The health care industry comprises many enterprises of hospitals, nursing homes, insurance companies, drug manufacturers, hospital supply and equipment companies, physicians, real estate and construction businesses, health systems consultants, and accounting companies and banks. Numerous other authors have explored the idea of health care as business since the 1970s. It is a concept that health care providers and caregivers are finally getting used to. Some believe that recent developments in health care are a challenge to authority, autonomy, and legitimacy for physicians. The dominant interest groups in health care—government, employers, the public, and major provider groups—cannot agree on how to change and improve the system. They are "unwilling to risk the strengths of our existing health care system. . . to remedy serious deficiencies." (Ginzberg, 1990). The health care industry as a whole has contributed greatly to improvements in the health status of the general population while protecting often conflicting vested interests. At the same time, the health care industry has strengthened and kept the private business sector intact. In the United States, the health care industry functions economically as a source of growth, accumulation of profit, investment opportunity, and employment (Harrington and Estes, 1994).

The health care industry today consists of numerous major components. These components are:

- hospitals
- nursing homes
- physicians
- home health agencies
- supply and equipment manufacturers
- drug companies
- insurance companies
- new managed care organizations (like HMOs, preferred provider organizations, and IPAs)

- specialized centers (like urgent care, surgery, dialysis, oncology)
- hospices
- nurses and other health care workers
- administrators, marketers, lawyers, and planners
- research entities
- **long-term care** management
- respite care
- independent living centers

With these many and differing components, it is clear that the health care industry has become a complex system. The structure of the industry changed significantly through the 1970s and 1980s. According to experts, some of those changes included:

- growth and consolidation of organizations
- integration across the continuum of care
- increase in private nonprofit and for-profit ownership of organizations
- diversification of services
- organizational restructuring (Harrington and Estes, 1994)

The industry became dominated by large hospital and managed care/ insurance organizations. Health care is no longer the province of individual hospitals and solo physician practitioners. There are now large corporate hospital systems overseeing large numbers of hospitals and multi-specialty or multiple-member physician practices, sometimes with multiple office sites.

Hospitals compose the largest sector of the health care industry. While the growth of hospital expenditures has increased rapidly, the number of community hospitals has actually declined (Harrington and Estes, 1994). Many of these closures were in small rural hospitals, but community hospitals also merged, leaving fewer individual hospital entities. The number of hospital beds began to decline in the late 1980s as well. This is primarily due to the focus on lowering hospital admissions and shortening lengths of stay. Beginning in the 1980s, hospitals shortened lengths of stay, reduced occupancy rates, and had a decline in admission rates (Harrington and Estes, 1994).

Although the number of community hospitals is dropping, the number of specialized hospitals is increasing. Large growth areas include facilities specializing in women's health, psychiatry, rehabilitation, and oncology care.

Nursing homes have also grown rapidly since the late 1980s. As the population of the United States ages, more nursing homes will be needed to keep pace with the expanding aging population. Home health care agencies have grown rapidly since the introduction of Medicare and Medicaid in 1965. Estimates of home care visits have tripled since 1990 (Harrington and Estes, 1994).

Newer and more influential forces in the health care industry are managed care organizations. These include health maintenance organizations (HMOs), **preferred provider organizations** (PPOs), and independent practice associations (IPAs). HMOs provide health care services on the basis of fixed-fee monthly charges per enrolled member.

Private health care insurance companies were one of the largest sectors of the health care industry. Many private insurance companies now offer their own managed care plans. As enrollments in HMOs and PPOs increase across the nation, it is anticipated that traditional indemnity insurance plan membership and coverage will continue to decline.

Physician practice arrangements have changed since the 1980s, moving to larger group practices and partnership arrangements. Because of this, physicians are continuing to develop larger and more complex forms of group practice. Physicians are also involved in the ownership and operations of health care business activities such as HMOs, PPOs, and **independent physician organizations** (IPOs).

Horizontal integration is another one of the major changes evident in health care. Horizontal integration means that hospitals have linked together their business functions under one corporate identity or system. This benefits hospitals because they can save money on operating facilities as well as share costs between the hospitals. Hospitals linked in this manner are called multi-hospital systems. The number of multi-hospital systems has increased 60 percent in the past 25 years, according to US Department of Commerce data from 1994.

Multi-hospital corporations are also consolidating, with large companies controlling the largest share of the overall hospital market. In 1990, the five largest nonprofit hospital systems controlled just under 20 percent of the nonprofit hospital beds, while the five largest for-profit hospital systems controlled almost 75 percent of the for-profit beds (Harrington and Estes, 1994). Much of the recent increase in multi-hospital systems is a result of the purchase or lease of existing facilities and the mergers of hospital organizations. Construction of new hospital facilities has not increased.

Vertical integration of organizations has also taken place. Vertical integration of hospitals and other entities means that organizations are formed that offer different levels and types of services under one organization. For example, the Tenet Healthcare organization owns hospitals, physician group practices, IPAs, and home care agencies. Catholic Healthcare West, a Western health care system, owns hospitals, physician groups, and an independent practice association with capitated enrollee lives (members).

In addition to traditional medical care, unconventional health therapies—those not usually taught in established medical and other professional schools—contribute significantly to the amount and cost of health care. It is estimated that one in three adults uses alternative forms of health interventions each year. It is also estimated that more visits are made to alternative care providers than to primary care physicians. It is estimated that over $10 billion per year is spent on such alternative forms of health care as yoga, chiropractic, relaxation techniques, therapeutic healing, megavitamins, and other mind/body techniques (Sultz and Young, 1997).

## HMOs AND MANAGED CARE

The experiences of the 1980s altered the way in which we think of health care in the United States. The experience of health maintenance organizations changed how health care is financed and delivered. It also blurred the lines between HMOs and other traditional insurance products and health care delivery. According to 1997 data, 75 percent of the population is enrolled in some type of managed care plan (McManis, 1993). Fifteen percent of the population is enrolled in established HMO plans (Hicks, 1994). The HMO industry grew and became significantly more visible in most areas of the country throughout the 1980s: HMO enrollment increased fourfold, from 9.1 million in mid-1980 to 36.5 million at the end of 1990 (Hicks, 1994).

The late 1980s were also a time of significant growth of other forms of managed care. In 1990, 33 percent of all insured employees were in either HMOs or PPOs. While no definite studies exist, changes involving adoption of what may be viewed as elements of HMO practice into traditional insurance would not have occurred without the example of competitive pressure generated by an increasingly visible HMO industry. The experience of HMOs encouraged the larger health systems to pay closer attention to the level and appropriateness of **inpatient utilization** and to the potential benefits of integrating financing with delivery to potentially exert influence over provider practice.

Throughout the 1980s, HMO provider networks tapped more heavily into more traditional medical practices and settings. Over half of all office-based physicians were affiliated with one or more HMOs in 1990 (Harrington and Estes, 1997). Network and independent practice association models, which base their provider networks on physicians in office-based **fee-for-service** practice, quadrupled between 1980 and 1990 (Harrington and Estes, 1997). Greater HMO penetration into fee-for-service practice also occurred with the growth in enrollment in prepaid group practice models. To some extent, these plans rely on office-based physicians to complement their regular full-time practitioners and to expand service areas and markets.

HMO ownership also grew and diversified during the 1980s. In 1980, the HMO industry was mainly based around independent plans devoted solely to the HMO business. Current HMO ownership reflects historical roots and considerable consolidation (Harrington and Estes, 1997). In 1990, insurers owned or managed 43 percent of all HMOs and enrolled 27 percent of all HMO enrollees (Harrington and Estes, 1997). In spite of considerable changes, the HMO industry still has strong roots in the past. Kaiser Foundation Health Plan remains dominant in the industry, representing 20 percent of optional HMO enrollment (Harrington and Estes, 1997). The majority of enrollees are in the largest plans with 100,000 or more members, such as Kaiser (Harrington and Estes, 1997).

The maturing HMO marketplace consolidation that took place in the early 1990s increased the share of stronger, more competitive plans. The HMO industry as a whole gained an estimated $38 billion in revenue in 1989 (Harrington and Estes, 1997). HMOs attribute their improved financial condition to increased revenues, largely due to premium increases and to improved cost controls, such as better **utilization review**, more efficient administration, and renegotiated provider contracts.

The most significant influence on the HMO industry is employers, who are responding to the rapid escalation in health care costs. If you thought it was insurance companies that caused managed care to be developed, guess again. Employers, particularly large ones, have become more involved purchasers, actively engaged in assessing the value of each benefit option and designing the total benefit package. Employers now request data on utilization, demographics, quality of care, costs, finances, and consumer satisfaction from HMO providers and plans. Employers are also becoming more assertive in influencing the structure and operations of HMOs.

The HMO industry expanded significantly in the 1980s and early 1990s. This resulted in a more geographically dispersed base of enrollees and a more diversified industry. Though most HMOs remain small and many are independent, the majority of enrollees are either in the largest plans (like Kaiser) or in plans sponsored by multi-HMO companies. Further consolidation over the next several years is likely to occur, due to variability of financial performance and market position across the industry.

Heavy regulations and health care policy legislation are also likely to escalate, due to a health care consumer backlash that started with vehemence in the early 1990s. More strict regulation and oversight for HMO plans is likely in the future as well. Despite the health care industry's diversity, HMOs continue to have unique properties such as an ability to absorb financial risk, comprehensive benefits, and integrated delivery systems with provider incentives to be more efficient. Although some of these properties have caused concern among enrollees, it is likely that HMOs and other managed care products will continue to form the backbone of the US health care system.

According to Sultz and Young, in their book *Healthcare USA* (1997), managed care refers to various arrangements that link health care financing and service delivery. It allows payers to exercise significant economic control over how and what services are delivered. Some of the common features found in managed care organizations (MCOs) include:

- provider panels: providers are selected to care for members
- limited choice: members must choose providers affiliated with the plan
- gatekeeping: members must obtain a referral for specialty or inpatient services
- risk sharing: providers share in the health plan's financial risk through capitation and other methods
- quality management and utilization review: the plan monitors provider practices and medical outcomes to identify deviations from

quality and efficiency standards set by the plan (Sultz and Young, 1997)

The government has enhanced anti-fraud enforcement tactics toward HMOs in the past few years. The enforcement strategies have targeted overbilling and overuse of services in fee-for-service arrangements. Recently, federal and state prosecutors have begun hunting for providers and plans that undertreat managed care patients. Some providers have already had cases filed and have agreed to large settlements.

Because of the data kept by doctors, hospitals, and health plans, it is apparently easy for prosecutors to pinpoint both over-utilization/over-billing and under-utilization. The Health Insurance Portability and Accountability Act of 1996 created funding for fraud detection, as did the Clinton administration's new fraud enforcement initiatives. In addition, both state and federal moves to further define and legislate the rights of consumers in managed care plans will lend clout to the prosecutors. Consumer protection rules are expected to assist prosecutors because they specify what plans are required to provide.

Hospitals, health plans, and physicians will all face increased scrutiny as more and more Medicare and Medicaid patients are served through managed care arrangements and as providers contract directly with Medicare to serve seniors in capitated plans. It is expected that as more beneficiaries of federal programs move into managed care, more whistle-blowers will emerge and cases will flow from that process.

Attorneys for health plans and providers argue that taking health systems to court for alleged under-treatment is misusing fraud statues. They believe this is a quality-of-care issue that should be addressed through existing regulations. The criminal or civil actions resulting from prosecutions would be based on the False Claims Act and other statutes. Prosecutors could be aided by whistle-blowers who are allowed to pocket up to a quarter of the damages.

The main organization behind health care fraud prosecution is the managed care fraud task force assembled by the Department of Justice and the Department of Health and Human Services' inspector general's office. The theory behind demonstrating managed care fraud is simple: Plans and providers say they will provide all medically necessary care and are paid up front to do so. If there is a scheme that results in denial of appropriate care, then both the government and the beneficiaries have been defrauded.

Plans may also be held liable for fraudulent actions by providers with whom they subcontract.

Health plans that use confidential criteria to deny coverage for requested services, then refuse to let doctors and patients talk with the review nurses who issue the denials, are an example of potential health care fraud, according to James Sheenan, an assistant US attorney in Philadelphia (Meyer, 1998). Other potential examples include **Medicare HMOs** that systematically disenroll sicker seniors and recruit healthier ones, fewer services provided to capitated patients than to those in the traditional indemnity plans, numerous complaints from doctors and patients, and excessive profits. Sheenan says, "We're looking at a volume of complaints about managed care, trying to figure out what is egregious behavior and what constitutes a pattern that shows intention or reckless conduct". He believes the biggest quality-of-care and under-treatment problems lie in behavioral health services, emergency care, and chronic care (1998).

Managed care fraud involves diverting prepaid fees from care delivery and results in patients' not getting the services or specialty referrals they need. Marketing, enrollment, and disenrollment are other likely areas for fraud prosecution. However, if providers and plans do away with all of the cost control mechanisms because they are afraid of fraud prosecution, everyone will pay more for health care. Providers and plans should not be at risk for fraud enforcement if they are ethical and honest.

## MEDICARE AND MEDICAID

In 1965, during the Lyndon Johnson administration, Title XVIII of the Social Security Act was legislated. The result of this legislation was the passage of Medicare, which provided the growing population of aging Americans with hospital and medical benefits. Essentially, in passing this legislation, the large group of elderly Americans, those over 65 years of age and most likely to need health care, were assured of hospital care that was paid for. Hospitals were pleased, because they were virtually guaranteed reimbursement for hospital expenses on the basis of "reasonable costs."

At the same time as the Medicare legislation, Title IX of the Social Security Act was also established. This program, Medicaid, was created as a companion program to Medicare. It was designed to support medical and health care needs of the medically indigent—those individuals without the means to obtain health care insurance or pay for their own medical care. The Medicaid program required all states to create joint federal-state programs that covered low-income individuals, including all those on welfare. The legislation was designed to give states broad options for determination of eligibility, benefits, and reimbursement rates. Because the state programs were run independently by each state, the programs differed widely.

Both Medicare and Medicaid had huge impacts on hospitalization rates in the United States. After 10 years of Medicare implementation, hospitalized patients over 65 years of age were spending twice as much time in the hospital as their younger counterparts, those between 45 and 64 years old (Sultz and Young, 1997). Medicare rates generally became the standards for establishing hospital reimbursement rates across the board. Because of this, Medicare did more to increase hospital expenses and increase health care costs than anything else.

In addition to fueling rising hospital costs, the Medicare and Medicaid programs also reduced the charitable role that many hospitals played in providing free medical care to those who could not pay for it. Therefore, hospitals became increasingly focused on profits, closing programs and services that did not produce enough revenues. The monetary incentives built into the Medicare system favored entrepreneurial, short-term financial interests in health care (Sultz and Young, 1997).

In the current health care environment of managed care, Medicare and Medicaid are being re-thought and re-vamped. Benefits have changed, and many reimbursable costs for medical care have been decreased. Co-payments and additional charges are now common for older patients. Many citizens eligible for Medicare are now being placed in HMO programs that receive capitated payments for care from Medicare. In addition, there are now **Medicare supplement policies** available specifically to the senior population (65 years and older) to cover medical expenses that Medicare sets limits on or does not reimburse for.

In some states, Medicaid has also entered the managed care marketplace. In California, for example, a pilot program was initiated in the mid-1990s that involved 12 counties in the state. This program was designed to place Medicaid patients into regular HMO plans operating in California. The goal was to decrease costs as well as eliminate patients using emergency services for routine medical care.

There were difficulties with the pilot program. Some of the problems involved complications from trying to transfer the immense number of medical records from Medicaid patients into HMO computer systems. There were also problems with patients being recruited by competing HMOs, up to and including patients receiving "sign-on" cash bonuses.

While the goal of using capitated payments was to decrease costs and enhance preventive care and screening, the implementation was problematic. However, the difficulties have been addressed and California is slowly moving all Medicaid patients (called Medi-Cal in California) over to HMO plans, a process called "mainstreaming" patients.

## DISCUSSION QUESTIONS

1. Describe the Medicare and Medicaid programs' features, benefits, and deficits.
2. Discuss the evolution of health care in the United States from the 1960s through the 1990s.
3. Define and describe HMO, PPO, MCO, IPA, PCP, and their respective roles in the changing health care system.

---

### BIBLIOGRAPHY

Aiken, L. et al. 1994. "Lower Medicare Mortality among a Set of Hospitals Known for Good Nursing Care." *Medical Care* 32(8): 771–785.

American Nurses' Association. 1993. *Nursing's Agenda for Health Care Reform.* Washington, D.C.: ANA Publishing.

———. 1994. *Every Patient Deserves a Nurse.* Brochure. Washington, D.C.: ANA Publishing.

———. 1996. *Registered Professional Nurses and Unlicensed Assistive Personnel.* 2nd ed. Washington, D.C.: ANA Publishing.

American Organization of Nurse Executives. 1996. *Talking Points on Hospital Redesign.* Washington, D.C.: American Organization of Nurse Executives.

Bathen, S. 1997. "The HMO Wars." *California Journal*, August, 12–18.

Bayley, E. et al. 1997. "Preparing to Change from Acute to Community Based Care." *Journal of Nursing Administration* 27:5.

Beckham, J.D. 1997a. "The Right Way to Integrate." *Healthcare Forum Journal*, July/August, 30–37.

———. 1997b. "The Beginning of the End for HMOs." Part 1. *Healthcare Forum Journal*, November/December, 44–47.

———. 1998. "The Beginning of the End for HMOs." Part 2. *Healthcare Forum Journal*, January/February, 52–55.

Bergman, R. 1993. "Quantum Leaps." *Hospitals and Health Networks*, 5 October, 28–35.

Bernard, L., and Walsh, M. 1996. *Leadership: The Key to Professionalization of Nursing*. New York: Mosby.

Beyers, M. 1996. "The Value of Nursing." *Hospitals and Health Networks*, 5 February, 52.

Brink, S. et al. 1997. "America's Top HMOs." *US News and World Report*, 13 October, 60–69.

Brock, R. 1996. "Head for Business." *Hospitals and Health Networks*, 5 December, 62–66.

Burda, D. 1994a. "A Profit by Any Other Name Would Still Give Hospitals the Fits." *Modern Healthcare*, 8 August, 115–136.

———. 1994b. "Layoffs Rise as Pace of Cost-Cutting Accelerates." *Modern Healthcare*, 12 December, 32.

———. 1995. "ANA Report Stokes Restructuring Debate." *Modern Healthcare*, 13 February, 38.

Burns, J. 1993. "Caring for the Community." *Modern Healthcare*, 8 November, 30–33.

Butts, J., and Brock, A. 1996. "Optimizing Nursing through Reorganization: Mandates for the New Millennium." *Nursing Connections* 9(4): 5–10.

California Nurses Association. Web Site Home Page. http://www.califnurses.org/

California Taxpayers Against Higher Health Costs. 1996. Ballot materials.

Christensen, P., and Bender, L. 1994. "Models of Nursing Care in a Changing Environment." *Orthopaedic Nursing* 13(2): 64–70.

Clarkson Hospital. 1995. "Patient Focused Care." Presentation handouts, June 1995, Omaha, Nebraska.

Coile, R. 1993a. "California Healthcare 2001: The Outlook for America's Bellwether State." *Hospital Strategy Report* 5(4), February, 1.

———. 1993b. "California Hospitals in the 21st Century." *California Hospitals*, November/December, 7–10.

———. 1994a. "Primary Care Networks: The Integrators of Care in an Integrated Delivery System." *Hospital Strategy Report* 6(8): 1–3.

———. 1994b. "Capitation: The New Food Chain of HMO Provider Payment." *Hospital Strategy Report* 6(9): 1–3.

Commonwealth Fund. 1995. *Healthcare Statistics*. Washington, D.C.: US Health Care Financing Administration.

Curran, C., ed. 1990. "IDN Core Competencies and Nursing's Role." *Nursing Economics*, December.

Davis, C., ed. 1996. *Nursing Staff in Hospitals and Nursing Homes: Is It Adequate?* National Institute of Medicine. Baltimore: National Academy Press.

Donaho, B., ed. 1996. *Celebrating the Journey: A Final Report on Strengthening Hospital Nursing*. Philadelphia: National Academy Press.

Dracup, K., and Bryan-Brown, C., eds. 1998. "Thinking Outside the Box and Other Resolutions." *American Journal of Critical-Care*, January, 1.

Eck, S. et al. 1997 "Consumerism, Nursing and the Reality of Resources." *Nursing Administration Quarterly* 12(3): 1–11.

Flower, J. 1997a. "Job Shift." *Healthcare Forum Journal*, January/February, 15–24.

———. 1997b. "The Age of Heretics." *Healthcare Forum Journal*, March/April, 34–39.

Fralicx, R., and Bolster, C.J. 1997. "Preventing Culture Shock." *Modern Healthcare*, 11 August, 50.

Gardener, J. 1998. "Medicare Meal Ticket." *Modern Healthcare*, 22 September, 36.

Ginzberg, E. 1990. "Healthcare Reform—Why So Slow?" *New England Journal of Medicine*, 1464–1465.

Goldsmith, J. 1993. "Driving the Nitroglycerin Truck," *Healthcare Forum Journal*, March/April, 36–44.

———. 1996. "Managed Care Mythology: Supply Dreams Die Hard." *Healthcare Forum Journal*, November/December, 43–47.

Golub, E. 1995. "Revisiting Our Ideas about Health." *Hospitals and Health Networks*, 20 January, 78.

Goodman, J. 1993. *Twenty Myths About National Health Insurance*. National Center for Policy Analysis, Dallas, Texas.

Gray, B.B. 1994a. "Twenty-First Century Hospital Embodies New Concept." *NurseWeek*, 1 April, 1.

———. 1994b. "Changing Skill Mix Reorders Healthcare Delivery System." *NurseWeek*, 2 December, 14.

———. 1995a. "Nurses Face Ethics of Rationing as Healthcare Industry Evolves." *NurseWeek*, 2 April, 20–22.

———. 1995b. "Issues at the Crossroads." Parts 1 and 2. *NurseWeek*, 1 October, 1.

Grayson, M., ed. 1995. "Clinical Maneuvers." *Hospitals and Health Networks*, 5 January, 52.

———. 1997. "Stuck on a Strategy." *Hospitals and Health Networks*, 5 October, 74–76.

Grimaldi, P. 1998. "PSO Requirements Taking Shape." *Nursing Management*, February, 14–18.

Hammers, M.A. 1994. "Crystal Ball Gazing with Leland Kaiser." *RN Times*, 5 September, 8–10.

Harrington, C., and Estes, C., eds. 1994. *Health Policy and Nursing*. 1st ed. Boston: Jones and Bartlett. 1997. *Health Policy and Nursing*. 2nd ed. Boston: Jones and Barlett.

Healthcare Advisory Board. 1992a. "Executive Report to the CEO: The Merits of Patient-Focused Care." Acetate presentation, October, The Advisory Board Company, Washington, D.C.

Healthcare Advisory Board. 1992b. "Toward a Twenty-First Century Hospital: Designing Patient Care." Acetate presentation, October, The Advisory Board Company, Washington, D.C.

Hicks, L. 1994. *Health Policy and Nursing*. New York: Mosby.

Katzenbaach, J.R., and Smith, D.K. 1993. *The Wisdom of Teams.* New York: Harper Collins.

Keepnews, D., and Marullo, G. 1996. "Policy Imperatives for Nursing in an Era of Healthcare Restructuring." *Nursing Administration Quarterly* 20(3):19–31 (spring).

Kunen, J. 1996. "The New Hands-Off Nursing." *Time,* 30 September, 55–57.

Lanara, V.A. 1993. "The Nurse of the Future, Role and Function." *Journal of Nursing Management* 1: 83–87.

Lumsdon, K. 1994a. "It's a Jungle Out There!" *Hospitals and Health Networks,* 20 May, 68–72.

———. 1994b. "Want to Save Millions?" *Hospitals and Health Networks,* 5 November, 24–32.

———. 1995a. "Watch for Flying Phrases." *Hospitals and Health Networks,* 20 March, 79–81.

———. 1995b. "Mean Streets." *Hospitals and Health Networks,* 5 October, 44–52.

———. 1995c. "Working Smarter, Not Harder." *Hospitals and Health Networks,* 5 November, 27–31.

———. 1995d. "Faded Glory." *Hospitals and Health Networks,* 5 December, 31–36.

MacStravic, S. 1997. "Managing Demand: The Wrong Paradigm." *Managed Care Quarterly* 5(4): 8–17.

Malone, B. et al. 1996. "A Grim Prognosis for Healthcare." *American Journal of Nursing Survey Results,* November, 40.

Manthey, M. 1994. "Issues in Patient Care Delivery." *Journal of Nursing Administration* 24(12): 14–16.

McCloskey, J., and Grace, H. 1997. *Current Issues in Nursing.* 5th ed. New York: Mosby.

McManis, G.L. 1993. "Reinventing the System." *Hospitals and Health Networks,* 5 October, 42–48.

Merisalo, L., ed. 1998a. "Investment in High-Tech Infrastructure Key to Future Success." *Managed Care Payment Advisor,* January, 1–2.

———. 1998b. "RN Staff Cuts Due to Managed Care Pressures May Be Costly." *Managed Care Payment Advisor,* March, 1–2.

Meyer, H. 1998. "Fraud Storm Surges Toward HMOs." *Hospitals and Health Networks,* 20 February, 28–29.

Miller, J. 1995. "Leading Nursing into the Future." *Harvard Nursing Research Institute Newsletter* 4(3): 5–7 (summer).

Moore, J.D., Jr. 1998. "What Downsizing." *Modern Healthcare,* 19 January, 12.

National Commission on Nursing Implementation Project, unpublished 1986–87 documents.

Olmos, D. 1997. "HMO Panel to Call for Consumer Protections." *Los Angeles Times,* 31 December, 1.

O'Rourke, M.W. 1996. "Who Holds the Keys to the Future of Healthcare?" *NurseWeek,* 8 January, 1.

Organization of Nurse Leaders. 1995. Focus Group Notes. *Nursing Issues*. 29 September.

Pew Health Professions Commission. 1995. "Healthy America: Practitioners for 2005." *Pew Health Professions Report*. Washington, D.C.: Pew Health Profession Commission.

―――. 1998. *"Pew Health Professions Report*. Washington, D.C.: Pew Health Profession Commission.

Pinto, C. et al. 1998. "Future Trends." *Modern Healthcare*, 5 January, 27–40.

Porter-O'Grady, T., ed. 1994a. *Implementing Shared Governance*. Chapter 7. New York: Mosby.

―――. 1994b. "Working with Consultants on a Redesign." *American Journal of Nursing*, October, 33–39.

Public Policy Institute of California. 1996. *Nursing Staff Trends in California Hospitals: 1977–1995*. October. Sacramento, California: Public Institute of California.

RN Special Advisory Committee. 1990. *Meeting the Immediate and Future Needs for Nursing in California*. Sacramento, California: State of California.

Sheehy, B. et al., 1995. "Don't Blink or You'll Miss It." *The Atlanta Consulting Group*, Atlanta, 69–87.

Shelton, K., ed. 1995. *Executive Excellence Magazine*, February.

Sherer, J. 1994a. "Job Shifts." *Hospitals and Health Networks*, 5 October, 64–68.

―――1994b. "Union Uprising: California Nurses React Aggressively to Work Redesign." *Hospitals and Health Networks*, 20 December, 36–38.

Shindul-Rothschild, J. et al. 1997. "Ten Keys to Quality Care." *American Journal of Nursing* 97(11): 35–43.

Shortell, S. et al. 1996. *Remaking Healthcare in America*. San Francisco: Jossey-Bass.

Shubert, D. 1996. "Hospitals Decrease Nurses' Role: Reassign Tasks to Aides." *Los Angeles Times*, 14 July.

Simmons, H. 1998. "The Forces That Impact Healthcare-Quality and Costs." *Healthcare Forum Journal*, January/February, 27–46.

St. Vincent Hospital. 1994. "CARE 2000: An Approach to Patient Focused Care." Presentation handouts, February 1994.

Sultz, H., and Young, K. 1997. *Healthcare USA*. Gaithersburg, Maryland: Aspen Publishers, Inc.

Teisberg, E. et al. 1994. "Making Competition in Health Care Work." *Harvard Business Review*, July/August, 131–141.

Truscott, J.P., and Churchill, G.M. 1995. "Patient Focused Care." *Nursing Policy Forum* 1(4): 5–12.

Turner, S.O. 1995. "Nurses: Are They the Key to Successful Capitation?" *Capitation and Medical Practice*, December, 1–2.

―――. 1996. "Capitation: Are You Ready for It?" *Surgical Services Management*, February, 43–45.

Udvarhelyi, I.S. et al. 1994. "Perspectives: Finding a Lasting Cure for US Healthcare." *Harvard Business Review*, September/October, 45–63.

Ummel, S. 1997. "Integration." *Healthcare Forum Journal*, March/April, 13–27.

Uustal, D.B. 1990. "The Ethical Challenges Raised in Managed Care and Integrated Care Environments." Lecture handouts, ONEC conference, February 1998.

# CHAPTER 4

# Changing Hospitals in a Changing Environment

If change occurs more rapidly outside an organization than inside an organization, that organization may be doomed to failure. Changes required for the emerging health care systems have been fast-paced and focused on survival. Many health care organizations are in chaos because they were not prepared for the velocity and breadth of change in the industry.

## A WORKPLACE IN TRANSITION

Many hospitals and health care providers are experiencing the uncomfortable results of downsizing and cost-cutting measures. Employees of hospitals and providers have difficulty coping with and meeting the challenges required in a changing environment. Major paradigm shifts are required for survival. (A paradigm is the way we think about a particular issue.)

Nursing has many paradigms that must change. Nurses are not prepared to change as rapidly as the environment is changing, but still must take an active role in planning their practice and function in the emerging health care system.

Nurses must focus on creating a new culture for the profession. However, past professional issues are now intertwined with emerging health care delivery issues. For instance, former issues like downsizing and lay-offs have led to more roles for registered nurses in the acute care setting, albeit with different functions. Nurses need to be prepared to be flexible in an ever-changing environment where hospitals and health care providers must experiment with different strategies in order to remain viable. Reengineering and redesign of organizational structure, systems, and work tasks; effective care management, including critical paths, patient-focused care models, and cost management related to capitated revenues for hospitals; sharing of financial risks and limiting resources are just a few of the new methods hospitals are devising to survive in the new environment.

Many nurses tend to focus on personal concerns, such as the lack of job security, risk of layoffs, and fears of cross-training, but some remain uneducated and uninformed about the national health care market, and naive about changes not directly affecting their current jobs. Among some staff, there is a perception that job options are limited for all health care personnel. This leads to feelings of victimization and a sense of betrayal because of changing nursing realities. Health care workers have lost the ability to control the marketplace and perks and face fierce job competition and a changing commitment of hospitals from providing jobs for employees to being competitive in the marketplace.

In fact, today there is an increase in alternative delivery sites that employ care providers other than hospital-based nurses. As a result, formal and on-the-job education for care providers is critical. Transition management, role change and expansion, and a need for new skills such as delegation, team building, and supervision of others are essential in this new marketplace. Analyses of most hospitals identify structures and systems that don't reflect the current health care environment of a system experiencing change. Many hospitals are still operating under the old model of care. These include a specialized care focus provided by department, such as postpartum or emergency care. There is often minimal interdepartmental communication and cooperation, causing fragmentation of care within the hospital and with other delivery sites. Cost-cutting measures have forced hospitals to reengineer and redesign organizations. In addition to flattening of the organizational structure, there is downsizing as well—at all organizational levels, especially middle management. Personnel have limited cross-training and flexibility; that leads to job insecurity and role confusion. There also has been some blending of previously specialized roles, like respiratory therapist or laboratory technologist, into interdisciplinary care tech and care partner roles.

Additional issues for hospital employees include feelings of powerlessness over their futures and loss of traditional job options. These feelings are often displayed in activities of employee militancy and union activism—two behaviors that usually result in polarizing employees against hospital administrators and limiting patient care options.

---

Changes in the health care industry have affected all providers, including physicians, nurses, administrators, technicians, etc. Some of the emotions and behaviors exhibited by staff in the midst of these changes include:

- fear
- anger
- sense of betrayal
- sense of loss
- defensiveness
- sense of entitlement
- limited flexibility
- "us versus them" mentality
- victimization
- denial
- perception of powerlessness
- narrow focus and tunnel vision
- limited marketability in new environment
- survivor guilt

---

Why are these emotions and behaviors being exhibited? What is happening? Some of the emotions may be attributable to ineffective communication within organizations. Constant, fast-paced change, and the uncertainty about change, causes the upheaval. These emotions and behaviors were previously found in the banking, aerospace, and airline industries. Unlike other industries, health care is in uncharted waters. Whereas jobs in other industries have been eliminated, job roles and functions in hospitals have changed, but many work tasks remain the same. Thus, hospital employees are in a new experience with limited knowledge about what the future holds. Because of uncertainty about the future, hospitals may be unwilling to spend money to assist employees to cope. There may be a lack of funds for employee education and a lack of transition management in hospital organizations. Pressure from managed care companies to be more cost-efficient may cause hospitals to become short-sighted in their vision and their planning for the future.

## SUCCESSFUL HOSPITAL ORGANIZATIONS' BENCHMARKS

As Harry Sultz and Kristina Young state in their book *Healthcare USA*, "The performance benchmarks of cost, quality, and access . . . have now become the survival criteria for the future" (Sultz and Young, 1997, 22).

Hospital care is now considered beneficial for its high technology but viewed negatively because of the corresponding high costs, inefficiency, and inequities. Stephen Shortell, in his book *Remaking Healthcare* (1996), discusses changes that hospitals must make to be both effective and efficient in the future. He summarizes these changes as:

- Become part of an integrated health care delivery system.
- Develop new management structures.
- Conduct population-based needs assessments (determine what community needs are in the service area).
- Create new relationships with physicians.
- Reengineer processes and systems, especially in clinical areas.
- Implement total quality management.
- Focus on outcomes, not on rewarding mere efforts.

Common characteristics of successful organizations seem to include flatter, non-hierarchical structures with more autonomous units. The staff produce high value-added goods and services while creating niche markets. Employees are quality-conscious, service-conscious, and quick to innovate. These organizations use highly trained, flexible people as the principal means of adding value. Facilities need regionalization, excellent clinical outcomes, satisfied patients, and a "winning look mentality" to be successful with managed care.

Hospitals will need to implement 10 steps to survive and succeed in the managed care marketplace, according to Donald L. Shubert, President of the National Institute for Medical Management Services in Camarillo, California. Mr. Shubert believes that successful organizations implement these steps, in varying order, to guarantee results.

### 1. Create a managed care strategic vision.

To begin the shift to a successful organization, the organizational culture and philosophy must be refocused to outcome-oriented managed care and capitated forms of payment. Implementation of changes must come from top executives who "walk the walk" and "talk the talk." Employees must take responsibility in their business and careers for the success of the overall organization.

### 2. Create a managed care strategic plan.

To create a managed care strategic plan, the vision must be complete. Strategic success will determine organizational redesign to achieve acceptable outcomes, cost reductions, coordinated care delivery, and patient satisfaction. The organization will need to involve employees who are visionary and capable of assisting with making changes. Strategically identify what the consumer expects from an integrated delivery system and create those programs and processes. Design an integrated, community-based health care delivery model focused on the continuum of care.

Organizations must also develop a transition management plan. This includes dealing with transition and accepting culture shock and the emotions and behaviors discussed previously. A communication plan must be designed to support the cost of mentoring employees and managers to get them through transition. Encourage and reward professional accountability among employees. Provide transition training and educational programs to realign skills for new system requirements.

### 3. Educate and communicate with all stakeholders in the integrated network.

The stakeholders in the integrated delivery network are all employees, volunteers, physicians, and trustees. Everyone who has a vested interest in the success of the organization is a stakeholder. Employees must be educated about managed care plans and systems to be able to work efficiently in and support them.

### 4. Create a physician contracting entity that will work with the hospital.

A physician contracting entity is a formal group of doctors who have a contract with the hospital and insurance companies to provide medical care to patients. Examples of physician contracting entities include independent physician organizations (IPOs) and **physician-hospital organizations** (PHOs). Creation of a separate organization to manage the work between physicians and hospitals is called a management services organization (MSO). Employees need to be educated about these entities and the organizations' roles and relationships with the hospital. Organizations must foster, encourage, and promote collaboration among physicians, employees, and physician contracting groups.

### 5. Obtain capitation contracts with risk sharing.

Risk sharing, risk pool contracting, or at-risk contracts reflect the hospital's participation in the financial risk of providing care because no one knows how much care will be delivered. If care costs more than the combined monies of hospital and physicians, then no one gets any profit. Risk sharing is considered a cornerstone in a successful capitation system because everyone has equal financial motivation to manage care effectively under fixed-fee, capitated contracts. Successful risk-sharing contracts create an environment that supports collaborative efforts in managing patient care. Nursing is vital to the success of a managed care system. Patient outcomes and payer satisfaction will make capitation successful. Nurses and other health care providers have critical roles in a managed care environment

### 6. Develop a total continuum of care.

A continuum of care is best described as all the services and programs available for patients regardless of age or disease. It is whatever services patients require throughout their lifetime. A continuum of care is critical because payers want to contract with networks who have the best quality outcomes and the most services available for patients. Nursing is essential to the development and function of the care continuum.

Care continuums focus on health promotion, prevention, and wellness. The goal is to minimize hospital admissions and maximize management of disease outside the hospital. The continuum will depend on involvement and coordination of other local agencies to support community health status. For example, a large percentage of recent high-risk deliveries within a hospital is concentrated in a geographic area known for poverty living standards. Other community agencies will be involved in trying to limit these high-risk deliveries. The department of building and safety will evaluate family living quarters. The sanitation department will address environmental improvement. Fire service will evaluate fire hazards. Police departments will assist in "cleaning up" the area by increasing patrols and arrests.

There are wonderful opportunities for nurses in expanded roles in community health clinics, home care management of high-risk patients, wellness programs, and parish nurse programs. Chronic diseases that are expensive for hospitals to manage, including chronic obstructive pulmonary disease, hypertension, and diabetes, will be managed outside hospitals in chronically ill group locations and clinics. Hospitals will directly provide or contract with local agencies to provide such disease management services as home care, **outpatient** surgical care, infusion care, and oncology clinics.

### 7. Develop the ability to manage care effectively.

Managing care means coordinating all care providers who deal with a given patient. It is critical to have administrative understanding of and commitment to creating and supporting an environment for managing care in a cost-effective, quality manner. There must be empowered nursing staff who accept responsibility and accountability for managing care. Nurses must be visionary and open-minded. With motivation and commitment to managing care, every care provider is accountable to give the best care in the most cost-efficient way.

Strategies for effective management include development of a clinical leadership model where nurses coordinate care and the fostering of collaboration between disciplines and departments. Nurses must participate in redesigning work at the task level and determining what is truly critical to patient care.

Critical paths and care maps can be used to coordinate care and document expected outcomes and deviations. These pathways need to be developed along the continuum of care, and not limited exclusively to the acute care setting. The purpose of critical paths and care maps is to provide guidelines, not to dictate care. The function of case managers is to help reduce lengths of stay to the fewest possible days. Patients' status is actively monitored as is their potential to be managed successfully outside the hospital by modalities such as home care, infusion centers, and skilled nursing facilities.

Care and cost information about patients can be shared freely along the continuum while confidentiality is maintained on an ongoing, centralized basis. Information-sharing facilitates both timely decision making and effective use of resources. The resulting patient-focused care can also reduce the cost of care and increase care quality.

Multifaceted and cross-trained caregivers provide not only cost-effective care, but improved patient satisfaction. The more flexible an employee is, the more valuable that employee will be. There will be fewer inpatient admissions and reduced cash flow; therefore, fewer employees who can do more are needed. Staff who are cross-trained in a nontraditional manner (such as acute care nurses trained for home health) are extremely valuable to their organizations. Documentation of effective care management and outcomes will significantly change nursing charting; for instance, "appears to be sleeping" will no longer be acceptable. The California Nursing Outcomes Coalition (Cal NOC) project in California is one attempt to quantify and qualify successful patient outcomes.

### 8. Develop the ability to effectively manage costs.

Risk-sharing contracts is one way hospitals participate in cost management. A risk-sharing contract means that everyone involved with a patient—the physicians, hospital, clinics, and payers—shares in the financial risks and rewards of providing care. In the traditional health care system, the insurance company carried all of the financial risk for patient care costs. Although hospitals purchased expensive, highly technical equipment, they were not at risk for nonpayment if care costs escalated or if a patient developed complications.

Consideration of lower-cost care options outside the hospital are a vital part of cost management. Effective **case management** of hospital utilization combined with effective alternative care delivery is vital to controlling care costs as well as to ensuring care quality. Critical path care management, effective case management, and using alternatives to hospitalization are all-important strategies for managing costs. Cost management is a significant commitment that hospitals must make to remain successful in the managed care environment.

### 9. Develop integrated information management capability.

Management of information in hospitals has been an ongoing challenge. Providing correct patient care information to providers in a timely and convenient way while maintaining confidentiality is a difficult process. As the health care system changes, providing information outside hospital walls and interfacing across the care continuum raises difficult implementation questions. Managers of information need to create user-friendly information systems, with easy access requiring minimal skills. Patient information must be contained in a unified, integrated data management system conveniently accessible to numerous providers in different locations.

### *10. Develop capability to change the organization to meet the rapidly changing needs and environment of health care.*

Health care organizations must be flexible to be successful in this ever-changing environment. Transition and change must be managed within an organization so that employees can continue functioning productively. Hospitals must manage organizational transition to allow successful recovery of the organization and the ability to be open and flexible for the next cycle of change. Transition without management of the changes will have unintended side effects, such as: survivor guilt, cynicism, sense of betrayal, distrust, lay-offs of the wrong people, or overuse of consultants. Organizational recovery after transition must occur for the organization to remain vital and productive. Revitalization is critical to the future success of the organization. Nurses must be innovative and involved in creating the emerging system.

Employees must realize that change is the new way of life and that fear and uncertainty are normal reactions. Health care facilities in all areas must create a new culture of awareness, acceptance, and education. Nurses must have personal and professional accountability for the changes in their professional role and functions. In addition, nursing students must be educated about the need for change and the evolution of the nurse's role.

### IS YOUR ORGANIZATION MANAGED CARE–FRIENDLY?

Many organizations are already involved with managed care but do not have systems in place to support that method of health care delivery. Use the *Managed Care Readiness Assessment Tool©* that appears in Appendix A to assess your organization's readiness. You may want to replicate this checklist to use in your organization. After you complete the checklist, you can then determine your plan to implement managed care successfully.

## DISCUSSION QUESTIONS

1. Identify the components of the traditional health care system that no longer exist in your geographic area. Also identify and define the key components of the new health care system in your geographic area.
2. List and explain the components of the new health care system that are most important to 1) health care providers, 2) consumers, 3) nurses, 4) physicians, and 5) payers. Why they are important?
3. What components need to be more developed in health care delivery in your geographic area? Why?

### BIBLIOGRAPHY

American Nurses' Association. 1993. *Nursing's Agenda for Health Care Reform*. Washington, D.C.: ANA Publishing.

———. 1994. *Every Patient Deserves a Nurse*. Brochure. Washington, D.C.: ANA Publishing.

———. 1996. *Registered Professional Nurses and Unlicensed Assistive Personnel*. 2nd ed. Washington, D.C.: ANA Publishing.

American Organization of Nurse Executives. 1996. *Talking Points on Hospital Redesign*. Washington, D.C.: American Organization of Nurse Executives.

Ashton, J., and Fike, R., eds. 1996. *Reengineering for Patient-Focused Care*. Boston: Prescott Publishing.

Bayley, E. et al. 1997. "Preparing to Change from Acute to Community Based Care." *Journal of Nursing Administration* 27:5.

Beckham, J.D. 1997. "The Right Way to Integrate." *Healthcare Forum Journal*, July/August, 30–37.

Bergman, R. 1993. "Quantum Leaps." *Hospitals and Health Networks*, 5 October, 28–35.

———. 1994. "Reengineering Health Care." *Hospitals and Health Networks*, 5 February, 24–30.

Beyers, M. 1996. "The Value of Nursing." *Hospitals and Health Networks*, 5 February, 52.

Brink, S. et al. 1997. "America's Top HMOs." *US News and World Report*, 13 October, 60–69.

Brock, R. 1996. "Head for Business." *Hospitals and Health Networks*, 5 December, 62–66.

Burda, D. 1994a. "A Profit by Any Other Name Would Still Give Hospitals the Fits." *Modern Healthcare*, 8 August, 115–136.

———. 1994b. "Layoffs Rise as Pace of Cost-Cutting Accelerates." *Modern Healthcare*, 12 December, 32.

———. 1995. "ANA Report Stokes Restructuring Debate." *Modern Healthcare*, 13 February, 38.

Burns, J. 1993. "Caring for the Community." *Modern Healthcare,* 8 November, 30–33.

Butts, J., and Brock, A. 1996. "Optimizing Nursing through Reorganization: Mandates for the New Millennium." *Nursing Connections* 9(4), 49–58.

Byrne, J. 1993. "The Horizontal Corporation." *Business Week,* 20 December, 76–81.

California Strategic Planning Committee for Nursing. 1996. *Final Report,* August. Irvine, California: California Strategic Planning Committee for Nursing.

California Taxpayers Against Higher Health Costs. 1996. Ballot materials.

Chriss, L. 1996. "Nurses Learn How to Work with Assistants." *NurseWeek,* 30 September, 1–3.

Christensen, P., and Bender, L. 1994. "Models of Nursing Care in a Changing Environment." *Orthopaedic Nursing* 13(2): 64–70.

Clarkson Hospital. 1995. "Patient Focused Care." Presentation handouts, June 1995, Omaha, Nebraska.

Coile, R. 1993a. "California Healthcare 2001: The Outlook for America's Bellwether State." *Hospital Strategy Report* 5(4), February.

———. 1993b. "California Hospitals in the 21st Century." *California Hospitals,* November/December, 7–10.

———. 1994a. "Primary Care Networks: The Integrators of Care in an Integrated Delivery System." *Hospital Strategy Report* 6(8): 1–3.

———. 1994b. "Capitation: The New Food Chain of HMO Provider Payment." *Hospital Strategy Report* 6(9): 1–3.

Commonwealth Fund. 1995. *Healthcare Statistics.* Washington, D.C.: US Health Care Financing Administration.

Conti, R. 1996. "Nurse Case Manager Roles: Implications for Practice." *Nursing Administration Quarterly* 21:1.

Curran, C., ed. 1990. "IDN Core Competencies and Nursing's Role." *Nursing Economics,* December.

Davis, C., ed. 1996. *Nursing Staff in Hospitals and Nursing Homes: Is it Adequate?* National Institute of Medicine. Philadelphia: National Academy Press.

Donaho, B., ed. 1996. *Celebrating the Journey: A Final Report on Strengthening Hospital Nursing.* Philadelphia: National Academy Press.

Dracup, K., and Bryan-Brown, C., eds. 1998. "Thinking Outside the Box and Other Resolutions." *American Journal of Critical-Care,* January, 1.

Eck, S. et al. 1996. "Consumerism, Nursing and the Reality of Resources." *Nursing Administration Quarterly* 12(3): 1–11.

Flower, J. 1997a. "Job Shift." *Healthcare Forum Journal,* January/February, 15–24.

———. 1997b. "The Age of Heretics." *Healthcare Forum Journal,* March/April, 34–39.

Gardener, J. 1998. "Medicare Meal Ticket." *Modern Healthcare,* 22 September, 36.

Goldsmith, J. 1993. "Driving the Nitroglycerin Truck." *Healthcare Forum Journal,* March/April, 36–44.

————. 1996. "Managed Care Mythology: Supply Dreams Die Hard." *Healthcare Forum Journal*, November/December, 43–47.

Golub, E. 1995. "Revisiting Our Ideas about Health." *Hospitals and Health Networks*, 20 January, 78.

Goodman, J. 1993. *Twenty Myths about National Health Insurance.* National Center for Policy Analysis, Dallas, Texas.

Goss, T. et al. 1993. "Risking the Present for a Powerful Future." *Harvard Business Review*, November/December, 98–108.

Gray, B.B. 1994a. "Twenty-First Century Hospital Embodies New Concept." *NurseWeek*, 1 April, 1.

————. 1994b. "Changing Skill Mix Reorders Healthcare Delivery System." *NurseWeek*, 2 December, 14.

————. 1995a. "Nurses Face Ethics of Rationing as Healthcare Industry Evolves." *NurseWeek*, 2 April, 20–22.

————. 1995b. "Issues at the Crossroads." Parts 1 and 2. *NurseWeek*, 1 October, 1.

Groves, M. 1996. "Life After Layoffs." *Los Angeles Times*, 25 March, 3.

Hammers, M.A. 1994. "Crystal Ball Gazing with Leland Kaiser." *RN Times*, 5 September, 8–10.

Harrington, C., and Estes, C., eds. 1997. *Health Policy and Nursing.* 2nd ed. Boston: Jones and Barlett.

Healthcare Advisory Board. 1992a. "Executive Report to the CEO: The Merits of Patient-Focused Care." Acetate presentation, October, The Advisory Board Company, Washington, D.C.

Healthcare Advisory Board. 1992b. "Toward a Twenty-First Century Hospital: Designing Patient Care." Acetate presentation, October, The Advisory Board Company, Washington, D.C.

Hirsch, G. 1997. "Fit to be Tried." *Hospitals and Health Networks*, 5 November, 50–54.

Izzo, J. 1998. "The Changing Values of Workers." *Healthcare Forum Journal*, May/June, 62–65.

Keepnews, D., and Marullo, G. 1996. "Policy Imperatives for Nursing in an Era of Healthcare Restructuring." *Nursing Administration Quarterly* 20(3): 19–31 (spring).

Kertesz, L. 1997. "What's Right, Wrong?" *Modern Healthcare*, 11 August, 70–74.

Kunen, J. 1996. "The New Hands-Off Nursing." *Time*, 30 September, 55–57.

Lanara, V.A. 1993. "The Nurse of the Future, Role and Function." *Journal of Nursing Management* 1: 83–87.

Lumsdon, K. 1994. "It's a Jungle Out There!" *Hospitals and Health Networks*, 20 May, 68–72.

————. 1995a. "Mean Streets." *Hospitals and Health Networks*, 5 October, 44–52.

————. 1995b. "Working Smarter, Not Harder." *Hospitals and Health Networks*, 5 November, 27–31.

————. 1995c. "Faded Glory." *Hospitals and Health Networks*, 5 December, 31–36.

MacStravic, S. 1988. "Outcome Marketing in Healthcare." *Healthcare Management Review* 13(2): 53–59.

———. 1997. "Managing Demand: The Wrong Paradigm." *Managed Care Quarterly* 5(4): 8–17.

Malone, B. et al. 1996. "A Grim Prognosis for Healthcare." *American Journal of Nursing Survey Results*, November, 40.

Manthey, M. 1994. "Issues in Patient Care Delivery." *Journal of Nursing Administration* 24(12): 14–16.

Morrell, J. 1995. "Turn Your Focus Outside In." *Hospitals and Health Networks*, 5 December, 66.

McCloskey, J., and Grace, H. 1997. *Current Issues in Nursing.* 5th ed. New York: Mosby.

McManis, G.L. 1993. "Reinventing the System." *Hospitals and Health Networks*, 5 October, 42–48.

Merisalo, L., ed. 1998a. "Investment in High-Tech Infrastructure Key to Future Success." *Managed Care Payment Advisor*, January, 1–2.

———. 1998b. "RN Staff Cuts Due to Managed Care Pressures May Be Costly." *Managed Care Payment Advisor*, March, 1–2.

Miller, J. 1995. "Leading Nursing into the Future." *Harvard Nursing Research Institute Newsletter* 4(3): 5–7 (summer).

Moore, J.D., Jr. 1998. "What Downsizing." *Modern Healthcare*, 19 January, 12.

Olmos, D. 1997. "HMO Panel to Call for Consumer Protections." *Los Angeles Times*, 31 December, 1.

O'Rourke, M.W. 1996. "Who Holds the Keys to the Future of Healthcare?" *NurseWeek*, 8 January, 1.

Organization of Nurse Leaders. 1995. Focus Group Notes. *Nursing Issues,* 29 September.

Pew Health Professions Commission. 1995. "Healthy America: Practitioners for 2005." *Pew Health Professions Report*. Washington, D.C.: Pew Health Profession Commission.

———. 1998. *Pew Health Professions Report*. Washington, D.C.: Pew Health Professions Commission.

Pinto, C. et al. 1998. "Future Trends." *Modern Healthcare*, 5 January, 27–40.

Porter-O'Grady, T. 1994. "Working with Consultants on a Redesign." *American Journal of Nursing,* October, 33–39.

Public Policy Institute of California. 1996. *Nursing Staff Trends in California Hospitals: 1977–1995*. October. Sacramento, California: Public Policy Institute of California.

Rich, P.L. 1995. "Working with Nursing Assistants: Becoming a Team." *Nursing 95*, May, 100–103.

RN Scope of Practice, California Business and Professions Code, sec. 2725.

RN Special Advisory Committee. 1990. *Meeting the Immediate and Future Needs for Nursing in California*. Sacramento, California: State of California.

Sherer, J. 1994a. "Corporate Cultures." *Hospitals and Health Networks*, 5 May, 20–27.

———. 1994b. "Job Shifts." *Hospitals and Health Networks*, 5 October, 64–68.

————. 1994c. "Union Uprising: California Nurses React Aggressively to Work Redesign." *Hospitals and Health Networks*, 20 December, 36–38.

————. 1995. "Tapping into Teams." *Hospitals and Health Networks*, 5 July, 32–35.

Shindul-Rothschild, J. et al. 1997. "Ten Keys to Quality Care." *American Journal of Nursing* 97(11): 35–43.

Shortell, S. et al. 1996. *Remaking Healthcare in America*. San Francisco: Jossey-Bass.

Simmons, H. 1998. "The Forces That Impact Healthcare—Quality and Costs." *Healthcare Forum Journal*, January/February, 27–46.

Shubert, D. 1996. "Hospitals Decrease Nurses' Role: Reassign Tasks to Aides." *Los Angeles Times*, 14 July.

St. Vincent Hospital. 1994. "CARE 2000: An Approach to Patient Focused Care." Presentation handouts, February 1994.

Sultz, H., and Young, K. 1997. *Healthcare USA*. Gaithersburg, Maryland: Aspen Publishers, Inc.

Sund, J. et al. 1998. "Case Management in an Integrated Delivery System." *Nursing Management*, January, 24–32.

Teisberg, E. et al. 1994. "Making Competition in Health Care Work." *Harvard Business Review*, July/August, 131–141.

Truscott, J.P., and Churchill, G.M. 1995. "Patient Focused Care." *Nursing Policy Forum* 1(4): 5–12.

Udvarhelyi, I.S. et al. 1994. "Perspectives: Finding a Lasting Cure for US Healthcare." *Harvard Business Review*, September/October, 45–63.

Ummel, S. 1997. "Integration." *Healthcare Forum Journal*, March/April, 13–27.

## CHAPTER 5

# Nursing Care *Is* Managed Care

In many ways, managed care has become the public's dumping ground for everything that is wrong with health care. Health care consumers are full of anecdotal horror stories, citing the evils of managed care and MCOs. One of the stories heard over and over is that the cutting of registered nursing staff has decreased patient care quality.

As all providers deal with increased financial pressures in a managed care marketplace, reducing staff levels and changing staff mix is one of the first options considered by hospitals. Registered nurses are one of the highest paid professional-level staff groups, and labor costs compose about 60 percent of hospitals' total budget.

Cutting staff is the most common choice among hospitals dealing with the managed care financial squeeze. Registered nurses are eliminated, but at what expense? Does quality of patient care suffer? Does cutting RN staff really save money over the long term? Using fewer RNs doesn't automatically lower care quality, but hospitals have to be careful that by eliminating RNs they are not actually raising costs in the long term.

Cutting nursing staff has the potential to decrease care quality by increasing the likelihood that patients will need additional care. These patients may need to reenter the health system due to complications or relapse, and this adds to the costs of care and increases providers' financial risk.

For example, patients who don't receive physician instructions, or who are not provided with the education that enables them to understand and follow physician instructions, are at risk. These patients are likely to have problems that result in them ending up back in the health care delivery system. It is registered nurses who deliver the education and preventive care that stave off potential problems, such as post-discharge infections or recurring congestive heart failure. Nurses also do much more. They continually assess patient progress. They can facilitate outpatient services once patients are discharged from the hospital. Keeping nurses on staff may actually save money in the long run, although there are not yet a large number of studies that will prove it.

Nursing care is the backbone of managed care. Nursing has always emphasized education, prevention, early intervention, and care continuity, founding principles of managed care. When hospitals organize and manage patient care and use registered nursing staff to do so, they are improving quality of care as well as saving money.

Retaining nurses to perform nursing care, using nursing assessment and treatment skills, and overseeing the entire care delivery process during hospitalization can lead not only to cost-effective, higher quality care but to happier and more satisfied patients.

This *doesn't* mean that hospitals should go back to all-RN staff. Unlicensed assistive personnel (UAP) are fully competent when trained and closely supervised by RNs. UAPs can complement RN staffing. Activities like bathing, walking, and feeding can safely be done by UAPs. What nurses do need to continue doing themselves is to continually assess and monitor the patient, as well as to oversee, coordinate, and organize the plan of care. This planning, coordinating, and organizing also includes providing the post-discharge education needed by both patients and families.

What this *does* mean is that hospitals must cut staffing costs with caution. Even though payers will continue to limit reimbursement, it is up to providers to decide what costs to cut. They must carefully weigh cutting back on services that directly impact patient care. Hospitals must closely monitor their staffing changes, watching for potential patient problems or quality decreases. If their monitoring shows no negative patient outcomes, then the staffing changes they made are likely to be both safe and cost-effective.

Providers take on the responsibility to delivery cost-effective *and* high-quality health care when they accept managed care contracts. They cannot afford to compromise quality outcomes and patient satisfaction for the sake of the bottom line. It is important for cost effectiveness that patients discharged from hospitals are actually ready to and capable of continuing their care safely outside the hospital. Monitoring vital signs, evaluating symptoms, controlling pain, and educating patients and families are nursing functions that can enhance patient outcomes and eliminate duplicative costs from readmission.

Registered nurses lend quality and care value in other areas. Nurses can work in different sites of care as well. **Ambulatory care** services and physician practices also must closely examine the benefits and features that RNs bring to those care areas such as patient education and case management. Unlicensed and other certified personnel have widely varied training that is focused on learning tasks. Only RNs study theoretical and conceptual frameworks that allow them to develop unique nursing care plans using the nursing process for every patient they encounter. While cutting RN staff in these settings is tempting for the operating monies it initially saves, nursing practice and patient quality and satisfaction may be compromised in the long run.

There are some areas for hospitals to evaluate before they start eliminating patient care positions. In a recent article in *Managed Care Payment Advisor*, nurse consultant Anne Sherman recommended seven options for hospitals to consider before cutting staff (1998). While each hospital's situation is different, it is probably wise to evaluate care patterns and trends before blindly eliminating clinical positions.

Examine **diagnosis-related groups** (DRGs): What are the cost and revenue benefits from the DRGs most commonly seen at your facility? Are they high-volume areas to offset costs of providing the care? Are some DRGs a cost drain?

Control uncompensated care: Uncollectibles total an average of 5.7 percent of hospitals' charges. Of that percentage, charity care composes only 2 percent of uncollectibles. Bad debt accounts for the remaining 4 percent. Controlling bad debt is a method to enhance gross revenue by 4 percent.

Eliminate duplication: Evaluate patient processing systems to ensure that all patient information is completely and accurately collected during the pre-registration process. This will eliminate rebilling for wrong addresses or time spent trying to determine the correct patient employer. These types of redundancies cost a bundle.

Evaluate use of nurses: Nurses are valuable to health care providers. Ensure you are utilizing the role to enhance patient outcomes, improve care quality, and increase patient satisfaction. Don't get caught in the trap of replacing nurses with UAPs just because it is cheaper in the short run.

Use your nursing staff to manage care and provide disease management: Their follow-up will eliminate costly patient non-compliance problems and prevent reentry into the health care delivery system.

Focus on quality: Health care providers who focused solely on cost have learned the hard way to compete on a basis of quality, not price.

Assess patient needs: Patients will continue to enter acute care sicker and stay for shorter amounts of time. Maximizing patient monitoring and providing education prior to discharge can reduce relapses and readmission for patients (Sherman, 1998).

### SELF-MANAGEMENT IN MANAGED CARE

The ultimate goal of the managed care model of health care is to be able to limit use of services because patients have achieved better health. The theory is that if patients self-manage toward better health, they will use fewer expensive resources. Many patients can achieve better health if given guidance and education. Who is best able to give patients those tools to self-management? You guessed it: nurses.

Providers in the health care industry who bear financial risk for care have likely done as much as they can to eliminate excess costs from the system. Changing the service setting, discounting reimbursement, and shortening lengths of stay are valuable components of cost reduction and will continue to be used. However, those modalities are still based on an "illness model." Assisting patients with self-management is moving toward a true "wellness model."

With that idea in mind, improving patients' health is the next logical place to look for savings. Evaluating lifestyle choices and assisting with modification of non-compliant health behaviors such as obesity and smoking are areas where nurses can provide education, demonstrate healthier choices, and increase understanding. While using nurses in this type of role may not actually impact patients' negative lifestyle choices, it will enhance their understanding and leave the door open for potential changes.

Monitoring existing medical problems, assisting non-compliant patients, and verifying physician instructions are additional means to assist patients with self-managing their care, thereby reducing provider risk and potential expenses for medical services. Patients who would most likely benefit from this type of nursing intervention are chronically ill patients with complex medical problems. Newly diagnosed patients with chronic disease are also potential beneficiaries of this new approach to managing costs as well as care.

## WHAT ABOUT THE NEW NURSING SHORTAGE?

Reports in bellwether states like California are confirming providers' worst fears. Another nursing shortage is developing. This shortage currently seems limited to critical care skilled nursing staff, but the ever-increasing number of aging Americans coupled with the decrease predicted in nursing supply for the next century could spell disaster for providers down the road.

Many events in the world are cyclic. In nature, for example, the tides and hormonal patterns in animals and humans are cyclic and predictable. The cyclic nature of things we encounter helps us makes sense of circumstances while providing predictability in our lives.

Economic cycles are also evident but far less predictable in the United States. These cycles have affected nursing—especially critical care—profoundly. There were critical shortages of nurses in the mid-1980s, followed by layoffs and unit closures in the early 1990s. Patient care is an expensive commodity that is now being judged for value by cost.

Numerous nurses were replaced with UAPs. Twelve-hour shifts were eliminated, and overtime pay for the last four hours was canceled. Nurses had more patients to oversee and 30 percent less salary. Many felt powerless and at risk. The cycle has begun again. In California, there is a lack of critical care and emergency room nurses in metropolitan areas like San Francisco and Los Angeles. Both of these cities have documented their nursing shortages in local news articles (Dracup and Bryan-Brown, 1998).

MCOs and hospital administrators had predicted that fewer patients would require hospitalization and therefore there would be less need for nurses. They were wrong. The national rate of emergency room visits increased 9 percent from 1990 to 1995 (Dracup and Bryan-Brown, 1998). The reason for the increase is not clear, but earlier discharge and changing insurance coverage likely feed into the problem.

Options for nurses to deal with this trend require anticipating additional shortages as nurses age and retire and the demand for nurses across the country increases. Nurses can be proactive by employing several strategies. These strategies include:

- Return to school for further education. The message delivered by health care administrators is that the greatest opportunities in health care require bachelor's preparation.
- Assist with identifying successful retention and recruitment strategies for nurses. Issues like salary and benefit packages, tuition reimbursement, and child care must be addressed in a meaningful way.
- Proactively determine how to use UAPs safely. We will need more of them in hospitals as the nursing shortage worsens. We must determine training criteria, competencies, and safe task functions for them to perform.
- Work with hospitals to identify practices that benefit patients but are also cost-effective. Cost containment issues are not going away.

## DISCUSSION QUESTIONS

1. Identify the components of the traditional health care system that no longer exist in your geographic area, and identify and define the key components of the new health care system in your geographic area.
2. List and explain the new health care system components most important (and why they are most important) to health care providers, consumers, nurses, physicians, payers.
3. What components need to be more developed in health care delivery in your geographic area? Why?
4. Is there a nursing shortage in your geographic area? Of what type (e.g., in what specialty areas of nursing practice)? For how long?
5. What steps are being taken to deal with the nursing shortage? Are they helping? Why or why not?
6. How are potential nursing students being recruited in your area? Is it working? Why or why not?

---

**BIBLIOGRAPHY**

Aiken, L. et al. 1994. "Lower Medicare Mortality among a Set of Hospitals Known for Good Nursing Care." *Medical Care* 32(8), June, 771–785.

American Association of Ambulatory Care Nurses. *Standards for Ambulatory Care Nursing*. Unpublished report.

American Nurses' Association. 1993. *Nursing's Agenda for Health Care Reform*. Washington, D.C.: ANA Publishing.

————. 1994. *Every Patient Deserves a Nurse*. Brochure. Washington, D.C.: ANA Publishing.

Ashton, J., and Fike, R., eds. 1996. *Reengineering for Patient-Focused Care*. Boston: Prescott Publishing.

Beckham, J.D. 1997. "The Right Way to Integrate." *Healthcare Forum Journal*, July/August, 30–37.

Bergman, R. 1993. "Quantum Leaps." *Hospitals and Health Networks*, 5 October, 28–35.

————. 1994. "Reengineering Health Care." *Hospitals and Health Networks*, 5 February, 16–24.

Beyers, M. 1996. "The Value of Nursing." *Hospitals and Health Networks*, 5 February, 52.

Brock, R. 1996. "Head for Business." *Hospitals and Health Networks*, 5 December, 62–66.

Burns, J. 1993. "Caring for the Community." *Modern Healthcare*, 8 November, 30–33.

Byrne, J. 1993. "The Horizontal Corporation." *Business Week*, 20 December, 76–81.

Coile, R. 1994. "Primary Care Networks: The Integrators of Care in an Integrated Delivery System." *Hospital Strategy Report* 6(8): 1–3.

Conti, R. 1996. "Nurse Case Manager Roles: Implications for Practice." *Nursing Administration Quarterly* 21:1.

Curran, C., ed. 1990. "IDN Core Competencies and Nursing's Role." *Nursing Economics*, December.

Dracup, K., and Bryan-Brown, C., eds. 1998. "Thinking Outside the Box and Other Resolutions." *American Journal of Critical-Care*, January, 1.

Duck, J.D. 1993. "Managing Change: The Art of Balancing." *Harvard Business Review*, November/December, 109–118.

Eck, S. et al. 1997. "Consumerism, Nursing and the Reality of Resources." *Nursing Administration Quarterly* 12(3): 1–11.

Gray, B.B. 1994. "Twenty-First Century Hospital Embodies New Concept." *NurseWeek*, 1 April, 1.

————. 1995a. "Nurses Face Ethics of Rationing as Healthcare Industry Evolves." *NurseWeek*, 2 April, 20–22.

————. 1995b. "Issues at the Crossroads." Parts 1 and 2. *NurseWeek*, 1 October, 1.

Hagland, M. 1995. "Incent Me." *Hospitals and Health Networks*, 5 September, 7.

Hall, G. et al. 1993. "How to Make Reengineering Really Work." *Harvard Business Review*, November/December, 1191–131.

Healthcare Advisory Board. 1992. "Toward a Twenty-First Century Hospital: Designing Patient Care." Acetate presentation, October, The Advisory Board Company, Washington, D.C.

Hudson, T. 1997. "Ties That Bind." *Hospitals and Health Networks*, 5 March, 20–26.

Kanter, R.M. 1983. *The Change Masters*. New York: Simon and Schuster.

Lumsdon, K. 1994. "It's a Jungle Out There!" *Hospitals and Health Networks*, 20 May, 68–72.

———. 1995. "Working Smarter, Not Harder." *Hospitals and Health Networks*, 5 November, 27–31.

Morrell, J. 1995. "Turn Your Focus Outside In." *Hospitals and Health Networks*, 5 December, 66.

O'Rourke, M.W. 1996. "Who Holds the Keys to the Future of Healthcare?" *NurseWeek*, 8 January, 1.

Porter-O'Grady, T., ed. 1994. *Implementing Shared Governance*. Chapter 7. New York: Mosby.

Porter-O'Grady, T. 1994. "Working with Consultants on a Redesign." *American Journal of Nursing,* October, 33–39.

Shelton, K., ed. 1995. *Executive Excellence Magazine*, February.

Sherer, J. 1994a. "Corporate Cultures" *Hospitals and Health Networks*, 5 May, 20–27.

———. 1994b. "Job Shifts." *Hospitals and Health Networks*, 5 October, 64–68.

———. 1994c. "Union Uprising: California Nurses React Aggressively to Work Redesign." *Hospitals and Health Networks*, 20 December, 36–38.

———. 1995. "Tapping into Teams." *Hospitals and Health Networks*, 5 July, 32–35.

Sherman, A. 1998. "Nurses Key to Managed Care." *Managed Care Payment Advisor*, May/June, 98.

Shindul-Rothschild, J. et al. 1997. "Ten Keys to Quality Care." *American Journal of Nursing* 97(11): 35–43.

Shortell, S. et al. 1996. *Remaking Healthcare in America*. San Francisco: Jossey-Bass.

Simmons, H. 1998. "The Forces That Impact Healthcare-Quality and Costs." *Healthcare Forum Journal*, January/February, 27–46.

Stewart, T. 1993. "Reengineering: The Hot New Management Tool." *Fortune*, 23 August, 41–45.

Sund, J. et al. 1998. "Case Management in an Integrated Delivery System." *Nursing Management*, January, 24–32.

Teisberg, E. et al. 1994. "Making Competition in Health Care Work." *Harvard Business Review*, July/August, 131–141.

Turner, S.O. 1995. "Nurses: Are They the Key to Successful Capitation?" *Capitation and Medical Practice*, December, 1–2.

Ummel, S. 1997. "Integration." *Healthcare Forum Journal*, March/April, 13–27.

Uustal, D.B. 1990. "The Ethical Challenges Raised in Managed Care and Integrated Care Environments." Lecture handouts, ONEC conference, February 1998.

# CHAPTER 6

# Nursing Ethics in a Managed Care System

According to David C. Blake, PhD, JD, Executive Director of the Center for Healthcare Ethics at St. Joseph Health System in Orange, California, managed care causes both care providers and consumers to have questions about justice and fairness. The AMA Council on Ethical and Judicial Affairs states " . . . managed care can compromise the quality and integrity of the patient-physician relationship and reduce the quality of care received by patients." Clearly, to all involved in the health care arena—physicians, patients, nurses, legislators, and consumers—there are significant ethics dilemmas, issues, and concerns about our managed health care marketplace.

The ethics of nursing practice are also challenged in the managed care environment when payer expectations for pre-authorization approvals are in direct conflict with what a nurse believes and how a patient receives quality-based appropriate care. The core of our nursing souls and the very foundation of our practice are jarred daily by conflicts between patient care needs and managed care practices.

It's not that ethical dilemmas are new to health care or the practice of nursing. We have always had to deal with questions like "Should that patient with no evidence of brain activity be taken off the ventilator," and when nursing advocacy is required outside the hospital, we have been able to keep our patients safe when they are unable to advocate for themselves.

But we have never had to deal with such "in-your-face" ethical dilemmas as the ones now posed by the managed care environment, nor known such strain on the fundamental underpinnings and theoretical framework of our practice.

The old fee-for-service health care system also raised ethical dangers, but they seemed to be more related to the practice of medicine and physicians' frameworks than to nursing. There were conflicts of interest between providers and patients.

Treatment could be profit-motivated, as physicians were paid in relation to what and how much they did diagnostically.

Treatment now is motivated by what physicians are permitted or authorized to do by payers. This limits physician power to determine what is best for patient care, while at the same time it controls costs. One of the ethical dilemmas lies in whether the patient actually gets the best treatment if physicians are limited in the scope of medical service they can provide.

In the past, the individual physician was a medical entrepreneur. The result of physician entrepreneurship was a huge increase in lucrative specialties and subspecialties. There was also an increase in high-cost, high-technology medical therapy. Now, essentially, the physician is treated as an employee of payer plans, due to the payer's control over physician practice.

It was during the fee-for-service era of medicine that the rise of bioethics as a discipline occurred. This new discipline was the result of perceived abuses in medical research as well as changes in patient treatment in individual physician medical practices. Bioethics challenged the authority and paternalism of physicians. Issues of patient treatment and informed consent along with increasing empowerment of patients irrevocably changed the way physicians practiced medicine.

In addition, the reexamination of end-of-life treatment also enhanced the study of bioethics. The Robert Wood Johnson Foundation did studies in the early 1990s and discovered what it termed "a medical culture of 'over-treatment.'" The studies determined that patients and physicians were potentially incentivized by the fee-for-service system to avoid issues of justice and of mortality.

In his book *Three Realms of Managed Care* (1997), John Glaser talks about three entities affected by the managed care system: the individual, the organization, and society. Glaser believes there are questions of justice that exist in health care that affect individuals and communities alike. For example, do individuals owe any duty of consideration or concern for the needs of others in expecting or demanding health care, especially at the end of life? In states where health care of lower-income patients is funded by those employed, there have been intense discussions about the rights and privileges of health care related to social and financial class.

Another question the managed care system brings up is how important is the good of health care relative to all the other human goods that individuals need access to and that society needs to provide? Other human goods would include things like food and shelter provided by society for those individuals who are unable to provide for themselves.

From the individual patient perspective, there are both rights and duties for justice to be served, according to David C. Blake (1998). Do individual patients have ethical rights to what they want? Or only to what they need, as determined by others? Do patients have an ethical duty to give and take a fair share of health care goods? Take a fair share of health care when death is imminent? Or do individuals only deserve a fair share relative to society's other goods?

According to Blake, there are some important distinctions between health care and other human goods. Having health and receiving health care when sick or chronically ill are two entirely different states of being. In addition, there are significant cost differences between these two states. Preventive medicine to maintain health is a different and less costly commodity than the provision of curative medicine when one is ill. Public health measures, such as child immunizations at community clinics or diabetic screening for adults, are a different level of care than receiving sophisticated medical treatment.

Some critics argue that the practice of medicine and delivery of medical care is an economic commodity no different than any other important commodity such as food, clothing, or housing. These critics dismiss the notion of any type of de facto social contract in medical care. Others, including many physicians, would argue that medical care is a social good, not a commodity, and should not be affected by economic patterns of reality and change. This conflict has caused much debate and fostered changes. Health care is now becoming commercialized, and professionalism in medicine is giving way to a business methodology and more focused entrepreneurialism. The health care system is now widely regarded as an industry, and medical practice as a competitive business (Harrington and Estes, 1997).

To serve social justice, individuals must consider themselves potential health care consumers. In reality, just about everyone will use the health care system and services at some point in his or her lifetime. Potential patients must have reasonable expectations. They must be aware of the odds involved in lifestyle choices they make, such as smoking or consuming alcohol, and not always expect to beat those odds. In addition, potential health care customers must know the odds of medical care outcomes before they embark on obtaining the service.

Potential health care consumers must have a willingness to live with limits, especially when associated with choices for which we all bear some responsibility—for example, choices in employment and employee benefits or choices in political health care decisions. It is clear, as evidenced in all of our media, that not everyone is willing to be accountable for choices or to live with limits. The reality is that justice in a managed care setting likely includes all of us squarely facing our own human mortality, embracing our own death as an inevitable outcome, and perhaps even setting a "good death" as a priority goal in our health care system.

The application of economic theories and models to the health care system is becoming increasingly necessary and important, according to Lanis Hicks in *Health Policy and Nursing* (1994). As expenditures for health care services rose at alarming rates and policy makers developed cost-containment strategies, more economists and economic theories got involved (Hicks, 1994). No society, no matter how affluent, can provide all of its citizens with all of the health care and technology they might wish to consume. Since resources available to the health care system are limited, decisions must be made about who gets how many of these scarce resources. Consequently, a system must be developed for **rationing** available resources. Rationing is simply the distribution of scarce items by a system that "limits the quantity of product that can be purchased" (Hicks, 1994, p. 210).

At a societal level, nurses have always been concerned about the availability of health care to all individuals, regardless of ability to pay. This philosophy is adhered to in varying degrees by different professionals. To the extent that individual nurses have feelings about access to health services and managed care system structure, they will be concerned with public policy and health care practices at state, federal, and local levels.

Managed care is considered by many to be for-profit health care without regard to medical need or patient comfort. Managed care embraces concepts like clinical practice guidelines and outcome-based data collection. This means that payment to physicians and hospitals is not based on what potential benefit the patient may have had, but rather on the actual benefit that a patient demonstrates, as well as the potential odds for success.

Another ethical dilemma only now coming to light for MCOs is the emerging power of consumers/patients. For-profit HMOs are losing value in the stock market, and patients are finally speaking out about choice and quality (Brink, 1997). Providers apparently have finally realized that their target market is not the HMOs, but rather those whom the HMOs are hoping to insure.

Patients have become the true health care consumers. Their demands to regain provider choice have forced HMOs to open restrictive plans to retain market share. Enrollment in **point-of-service** (POS) plans skyrocketed in 1998. That eliminates HMOs' ability to limit patient access to providers. HMOs can no longer trade patients for price concessions and control of utilization. HMOs have opened to more providers and reduced cost control; this was mandated as a result of hospitals and physicians marketing their services directly to consumers.

This increase in HMO flexibility reflects our society of increasingly older, more affluent, and more educated consumers taking charge of their own health care. Sources like the Internet, medical media coverage, and the proliferation of medical information—normally accessed only by clinicians—for average consumers has changed the health care landscape and given consumers most of the power. This new consumer control will force HMOs to manage health care instead of irritating providers and consumers.

This leads to a final question, for which there is no easy answer. What is managed care? Is it an inherently immoral or morally flawed system of delivering and financing health care based on profit and denial of access to care? Or is it a morally neutral system that could, if properly controlled and administered, give incentives to both patients and caregivers to squarely face the fundamental ethical realities about life, death, lifestyle choices, and the relative value of health care in our society?

Nurses need to determine for themselves the answers to the questions in this chapter. Each nurse needs to evaluate and set his or her own moral compass. Only then will nurses be able to practice nursing comfortably in our new health care environment.

## DISCUSSION QUESTIONS

1. Identify three to five ethical dilemmas created for nurses by managed health care delivery. Are there potential solutions? What are they?
2. List three strategies nurses could use to deal with ethical dilemmas caused by managed health care delivery in your geographic area.
3. Are there any areas of managed care that nurses should not be involved in? Why?

---

### BIBLIOGRAPHY

Aiken, L. et al. 1994. "Lower Medicare Mortality among a Set of Hospitals Known for Good Nursing Care." *Medical Care* 32(8), June, 771–785.

American Association of Critical-Care Nurses. 1996. "Decision Grid for Delegation." Staffing Tool Kit. Aliso Viejo, California: AACN Publishing.

American Nurses Association. 1985. *Code for Nurses*. Washington, D.C.: ANA Publishing.

———. 1993. *Nursing's Agenda for Health Care Reform*. Washington, D.C.: ANA Publishing.

———. 1994. *Every Patient Deserves a Nurse*. Brochure. Washington, D.C.: ANA Publishing.

———. 1996. *Registered Professional Nurses and Unlicensed Assistive Personnel*. 2nd ed. Washington, D.C.: ANA Publishing.

American Organization of Nurse Executives. 1996. *Talking Points on Hospital Redesign*. Washington, D.C.: American Organization of Nurse Executives.

Blake, D. 1998. "Managed Care and the Questions of Justice." Lecture handouts, ONEC conference, February 1998, San Diego, California.

Brink, S. et al. 1997. "America's Top HMOs." *US News and World Report*, 13 October, 60–69.

Davis, C., ed. 1996. *Nursing Staff in Hospitals and Nursing Homes: Is It Adequate?* National Institute of Medicine. Washington, D.C.: National Academy Press.

Glaser, J. 1997. *Three Realms of Managed Care*. San Francisco: Jossey-Bass.

Golub, E. 1995. "Revisiting Our Ideas about Health." *Hospitals and Health Networks*, 20 January, 78.

Gray, B.B. 1994a. "Twenty-First Century Hospital Embodies New Concept." *NurseWeek*, 1 April, 1.

———. 1994b. "Changing Skill Mix Reorders Healthcare Delivery System." *NurseWeek*, 2 December, 14.

———. 1995. "Nurses Face Ethics of Rationing as Healthcare Industry Evolves." *NurseWeek*, 2 April, 20–22.

Harrington, C., and Estes, C., eds. 1997. *Health Policy and Nursing.* 2nd ed. Boston: Jones and Barlett.

Hicks, L. 1994. *Health Policy and Nursing.* New York: Mosby.

Hirsch, G. 1997. "Fit to be Tried." *Hospitals and Health Networks,* 5 November, 50–54.

Keepnews, D., and Marullo, G. 1996. "Policy Imperatives for Nursing in an Era of Healthcare Restructuring." *Nursing Administration Quarterly* 20(3): 9–31 (spring).

Malone, B. et al. 1996. "A Grim Prognosis for Healthcare." *American Journal of Nursing Survey Results,* November, 40.

Manthey, M. 1994. "Issues in Patient Care Delivery." *Journal of Nursing Administration* 24(12): 14–16.

McCloskey, J., and Grace, H. 1997. *Current Issues in Nursing.* 5th ed. New York: Mosby.

McManis, G.L. 1993. "Reinventing the System." *Hospitals and Health Networks,* 5 October, 42–48.

Merisalo, L. 1998. "RN Staff Cuts Due to Managed Care Pressures May Be Costly." *Managed Care Payment Advisor,* March, 1–2.

Meyer, H. 1998. "Fraud Storm Surges Toward HMOs." *Hospitals and Health Networks,* 20 February, 28–29.

National Council of Nursing State Boards. 1995. "Delegation." *Issues 95* 15(1): 1–3.

———. 1997. "NCN Identifies Functional Abilities Essential for Nursing Practice." *Issues 97* 18(1): 8–9.

O'Rourke, M.W. 1996. "Who Holds the Keys to the Future of Healthcare?" *NurseWeek,* 8 January, 1.

Organization of Nurse Leaders. 1995. Focus Group Notes. *Nursing Issues.* 29 September.

Rich, P.L. 1995. "Working with Nursing Assistants: Becoming a Team." *Nursing 95,* May, 100–103.

Shindul-Rothschild, J. et al. 1997. "Ten Keys to Quality Care." *American Journal of Nursing* 97(11): 35–43.

Shubert, D. 1996. "Hospitals Decrease Nurses' Role: Reassign Tasks to Aides." *Los Angeles Times,* 14 July.

Sund, J. et al. 1998. "Case Management in an Integrated Delivery System." *Nursing Management,* January, 24–32.

Ummel, S. 1997. "Integration." *Healthcare Forum Journal,* March/April, 13–27.

Uustal, D.B. 1990. "The Ethical Challenges Raised in Managed Care and Integrated Care Environments." Lecture handouts, ONEC conference, February 1998, San Diego, California.

# CHAPTER 7

# Reengineering Nursing

Reengineering was first introduced in the mid-1980s by Hammer and Champy. These reengineering gurus defined reengineering as "the fundamental rethinking and radical redesign of business processes to achieve dramatic improvements in critical, contemporary measures of performance, such as cost, quality, service and speed (Hammer and Champy, 1993, p. 32)." Reengineering is not about improving existing processes: it is about starting all over and inventing the future.

Reengineering in health care is aimed at producing significant changes to the systems associated with the delivery of patient care. Reengineering should be synonymous with reinvention and asks the question: "If I were to start this service or system all over again, what would it look like?" An underlying premise of reengineering is that business processes should be designed around related and interwoven tasks that together produce outcomes that fulfill customer needs. These customer-focused processes transcend traditional departmental boundaries.

Systems and processes in organizations don't operate in isolation. They are interrelated and integrated. Reengineering is a global approach and therefore will impact multiple areas and processes of the organization. Reengineering drives significant and radical change. Reengineering is about creating what doesn't yet exist. True reengineering begins with the future and works back to the present (McCloskey and Grace, 1997, p. 313). The process is highly creative, innovative, and outside traditional thinking.

Unfortunately, many hospitals did not utilize reengineering in a pure form. Most facilities focused on a reengineering byproduct—-expense reduction. In true reengineering, expense reduction is a side effect, caused by restructured systems that increase productivity and efficiency as well as customer satisfaction.

It appears that hospitals, panicked by the exponentially increasing discounts from MCOs and radically declining censuses in the early 1990s, went on a reengineering quest. Most were hell-bent to reduce costs, regardless of the impact on patient care or customer satisfaction. The first rounds of reengineering were easy. It was discovered that 45 steps to get a chest X-ray could be cut down to 12 and that duplication between departments could be easily eliminated. Chief financial officers and administrators cheered as they saw expenses fall.

Then, additional reengineering strategies begin. Brought in by big consulting firms, strategies like patient-focused care and modular nurse staffing were introduced. RN positions were eliminated. UAPs were hired, with widely varying training, job descriptions, and competency proficiencies. The perception seemed to be: if nursing personnel are the largest wage expense, then reducing that expense is logical.

What *didn't* happen is the evaluation of what nursing care is and what nursing provides in hospitals. In the chapter on managed care, the nursing focus on education, prevention, and managing chronic disease is discussed. For reasons unclear, these major functions of nurses were lost on hospital administrators and CFOs charged with eliminating "fluff." Somehow, the role of nurses in hospitals failed to be clarified or understood by those responsible for keeping it intact. It was never articulated to those responsible what nurses did, how they functioned, why they were important, or what they contributed to care quality, patient satisfaction, and improved clinical outcomes. As a profession, nursing got hammered by hospital administrators trying to deal with managed care. We nurses probably asked for it because we have never been able to articulate what it is we do for patients and why we make a crucial difference.

The bad news is that RN positions were eliminated by the thousands across the country. UAPs were used as substitutes for RN staff. Using UAPs is not inherently bad staffing strategy. The error was in assuming that UAPs can *replace* RNs rather than *assist* RNs.

Reengineering patient care in hospitals looked mainly at staffing models. The actual systems of administering patient care services were never really evaluated. Hospitals are based on an "illness" model. Most facilities did not go back to the drawing board and create a new hospital based on what patients, physicians, and payers needed—the equivalent of a round pink chessboard. Rather, most hospitals continued to move the same chess players around on the same square black-and-white chessboard. Then they wondered why patients were unhappy, physicians were irate, staff's morale plummeted, and expenses didn't change all that much.

Preparing health care organizations for a new cost-sensitive and quality-based environment requires administrators to involve front-line workers in every aspect of organizational planning. However, as hospital providers face growing pressure to consolidate functions and facilities, eliminate redundancy, and respond to managed care, there is a tendency for managers and administrators alike to focus on only the big picture. Focusing only on system-wide operational and financial concerns can neglect or minimize workers' desire for job security and a voice in the decision making.

One avenue used by workers who feel underappreciated is unionization. Recent polls show an increase both in the filing of petitions for union elections and in unions' success rate once elections are held (Burda, 1994a). Filings are cause for administrator concern, even if elections are not held, because data from the National Labor Relations Board show that union organizers continue to be more successful in health care settings than with industry overall (Burda, 1994a). For example, unions won 58.3 percent of all health care elections in 1993, compared with a 48 percent win rate for unions in all industries. In addition, unions' overall success rate in health care elections is rising. The overall health care election-win rate for 1993 compares with a rate of 55.2 percent in 1992. The union win rate in hospitals went up almost 10 percent from 45.5 percent to 53.1 percent in 1993 (Burda, 1994a).

Like most executives, front-line workers are worried about the future direction of the health care industry and fearful of government attempts to overhaul the system. Some hospitals are unilaterally changing work rules and eliminating flexible working hours, such as those that allowed nurses who worked two 12-hour shifts on the weekend to receive pay for 40 hours of work. Others are changing staffing patterns to allow more cross-training of employees and reducing benefit levels. One hospital even told registered nurses they would no longer be paid for their half-hour meal breaks.

These changes at hospitals are occurring just as a number of unions are targeting health care workers for organizing efforts. Recently, nurses at hospital facilities in California and the Midwest have held strikes to protest **floating** policies and staffing patterns. The actions were characterized as efforts to ensure quality patient care and protect their nursing licenses.

While one can argue about the value of nurses fighting change, hospital executives may find it prudent for employers to avoid situations that lead to costly and tense conflicts with staff. Executives can accomplish more by improving communications with employees than they can by fighting a battle against disgruntled staff. Some hospitals have started employee newsletters specifically to communicate to their staff how reengineering efforts will involve them. Even better are efforts to include representatives at all staffing levels in designing and implementing institution-wide changes.

The good news is that hospitals and MCOs alike are beginning to understand, and evaluate in dollars, the value that RNs bring to the patient care arena. Consumers have grabbed control of their health care options and are demanding choices that include components that nurses provide. Hospitals are beginning to realize that nurses add value and enhance patient care. That change in mindset will drastically alter the reengineering plans for the future. Nurses can be assured of a key role in the managed care marketplace in the new millennium.

## PATIENT-FOCUSED CARE: A REENGINEERING STRATEGY?

Hospitals have created several reengineering strategies, including patient-focused care. The concept of patient-focused care seems somewhat odd and redundant to most nurses because their care has always been patient-focused. Patient-focused care is the result of patient-focused work transformation. This is a restructuring strategy that combines both work redesign and reengineering techniques. Using this method allows facilities to continuously improve quality of care and enhance the efficiency of all types of resources within the delivery system.

Patient-focused care has been described as "a kaleidoscope turning, rearranging the mosaic like interconnections of people and processes that make up the modern hospital to form an entirely different pattern" (Truscott and Churchill, 1995, p. 6). This type of delivery system aims to improve customer satisfaction and quality of care while reducing cost.

Since its first implementation in 1989 at Florida's Lakeland Regional Medical Center, patient-focused care has been gaining popularity nationwide. Over the past five years, proponents have converted one or more units within health care facilities so that resources and personnel are organized around patients rather than around various specialized departments.

Hospitals must change the fundamental ways they operate and deliver care in order to reflect an approach focused on the patient. Such an approach allows institutions to provide efficient care and also maintain their competitive edge. Establishment of patient-focused care is an intense and complex process. This formidable task requires years of commitment, from the design stage to implementation through evaluation. Moreover, the dedication of all departments, including administration, is necessary for success. Mediocrity cannot be tolerated at any level.

Restructuring health care organizations requires making hard decisions about how to best meet the needs of patients while containing cost. In patient-focused hospitals, employees have the opportunity for increased responsibility and the authority to meet patient needs with established accountability for patient outcomes.

Because the changing dynamics of work groups, tasks, and skills will remain a challenge for an extended period of time, it is imperative that staff are able to voice concerns and feel comfortable in their new roles. Ongoing support and opportunities for open, honest dialogue are crucial to success.

Hospitals using the patient-focused care approach continually improve the quality of care and enhance efficiency by eliminating resource waste within the delivery system. For example, key elements such as pre-admission testing, discharge planning, and surgical and pharmacy services are being reengineered to support the new patient-focused environment. With such services moving closer to the bedside, all aspects of inpatient care delivery are being assessed as part of work redesign.

Institutional administrators may wonder whether this delivery system is the right one for these difficult times. Nursing leaders as well as staff nurses must also carefully consider their own willingness to direct or to participate in such a process. Can you help design a vision for professional nursing that embraces change? Do you have the commitment necessary for this type of long-term project? For optimal results, you and your colleagues must share a strong belief that even though every crisis period has a certain amount of risk involved, tremendous opportunity also abounds.

As more hospitals face the challenge of remaining profitable in light of increased competition, declining resources, and revenue reductions, it is clear that they can no longer use traditional cost-control methods to survive in the health care marketplace. By changing the fundamental ways they operate and deliver care to reflect a patient-focused approach, however, institutions can not only focus on quality, but streamline operations. This increased efficiency also reduces duplication and enhances "seamless" care delivery.

Patient-focused care, as an outcome of inpatient hospital restructuring, requires significant organizational changes. For example, traditional hospital departments, structured as virtually independent "silos," must be realigned so that patient needs, rather than the department preference, are the focus of services. In turn, these services should be brought to patients whenever possible, instead of taking the patient to the service. Therefore, executive leadership must be open to review and readjustment as the process completes the full cycle.

Before beginning the restructuring process that is to result in patient-focused care, the organization must have a sound, clear vision. Without this critical element, it cannot remain effectively centered during the difficult transition period that will follow. Hospitals must restrain themselves from "jumping in and doing something quick," without a vision and an idea of where they are going. Moreover, without a vision, inappropriate compromises can result in less than optimal outcomes for the institution.

A critical step in the early part of the restructuring process is the selection of internal staff who will guide the teams and provide support. It is imperative that these key individuals are credible leaders across disciplines and have strong group process skills. These individuals need to believe in and share the organization's vision. Depending on the time frame allotted for results, some institutions also may use consultants to drive the process more rapidly or to provide an additional resource for change management. Together, these individuals, along with senior administrators, will help to revamp the highly compartmentalized organizational structure of the facility, moving services closer to the bedside and reducing the number of care providers interacting with each patient.

Traditionally, hospitals have had discrete, function-based services such as housekeeping, pharmacy, and laboratory. Unfortunately, this specialization has led to more fragmented, costly care and less than ideal customer service. For example, during a typical three-to-four-day inpatient stay in a large hospital, a patient may interact with 50 to 60 employees in numerous job classifications. In addition, the traditional hospital care delivery system reflects the needs and conveniences of the provider, not the needs of the patient.

This compartmentalization breeds process complexity and raises costs. Hospitals using a patient-focused approach have redeployed clinical, administrative, and support services to patient units from central departments. A primary goal of the patient-focused design is to provide at least 70 percent of all services on the patient unit (Truscott and Churchill, 1995). Only those services that have expensive equipment or highly skilled personnel remain centrally located. To achieve this objective efficiently, patient-focused units typically are larger than average and contain homogeneous patient populations.

## THE COMPONENTS OF RESTRUCTURING

A major element of restructuring is called process reengineering. This concept makes breakthrough changes in the systems associated with the delivery of care so that services are aligned with patient needs. Besides this gain in customer service, however, reengineering aims to improve measures of performance, including profitability, market share, and cost reductions.

Teams working on process reengineering usually are composed of information management staff, who understand the institution's systems and technology, and specially trained hospital employees, called process experts. These teams consider options and weigh alternatives carefully.

Process reengineering is not "bandaiding" the existing system so that it works better. Rather, it is a radical redesign resulting in a completely new system. Team members starting the project do not know what the final result will be. A common approach is to answer the question, "If we could start from scratch, how would we do this?" Also, according to Timothy Porter-O'Grady, "the best time to begin reengineering is when an organization is still doing well and has time and resources to commit to it" (Truscott and Churchill, 1995, p. 11).

Like total quality management and continuous quality improvement, reengineering analyzes the way an organization does business while identifying opportunities for improvement. Often, when reengineering ends, total quality management can be used to continue the process.

Reengineering is about major breakthroughs and radical, dramatic changes that provide significant gains quickly, within six to 12 months. It examines existing processes and cuts across boundaries while discarding the old process. It takes about eight to 10 weeks to design a new process, and several years to truly reengineer a hospital. It is a periodic rather than continuous process. There is greater emphasis on improving performance, profitability, and market share. Cost reduction is a side effect, not a goal or outcome focus.

Total quality management is a continuous process improvement, making small incremental gains over time. It focuses on existing processes. Total quality management takes a long time and is continuous. It focuses on customer satisfaction. Cost reduction is a side effect here, too, rather than a goal or outcome focus.

Another component of restructuring—work redesign—is often a difficult organizational change because it directly involves people and their jobs. Focusing on the question of "who does what?" this procedure requires a careful examination of patient care needs and the types of jobs that will most effectively and efficiently meet those requirements. Although work redesign models vary from institution to institution and across services, patient-focused care units most often contain cross-trained personnel, self-managed work teams, and empowered, accountable staff.

Cross-training usually includes four broad categories of generalists: professional, clinical/technical, support, and administrative. The professional category includes registered nurses, physicians, occupational therapists, clinical dietitians, and social workers. A clinical/technical generalist may be a respiratory therapist, an electrocardiogram technician, or a nonprofessional trained to perform a variety of clinical skills (such as phlebotomy, basic nursing care, and respiratory or physical therapy procedures). On the other hand, a support generalist assumes the more non-clinical tasks, like housekeeping, dietary, supply management, and transport, and an administrative generalist is involved with admissions, insurance verification, coding, completion of medical records, and unit secretarial duties.

The goal of cross-training is to decrease the number of caregivers who interact with patients. On patient-focused units, clinical generalists are cross-trained to meet most of a patient's needs. Additionally, any skill that is cross-trained requires that competency be established and then maintained through ongoing assessment and education. While this technique can produce role ambiguity and a loss of professional identity, it is not a single skill or set of skills that makes a professional. It is the unique combination of skills, knowledge, and abilities.

Besides cross-trained providers, patient-focused units rely on multidisciplinary teams to consistently work with the same physicians and care for similar types of patients. Both the specific number and mix of individuals on a team vary from hospital to hospital and must be carefully analyzed based on the needs of patients and the ability and expertise of professional and technical staff.

Similarly, the role of the nurse may vary substantially between patient-focused units and institutions. Work redesign consistently alters the role of the professional nurse and increases the need for registered nurses to be skilled in managing different levels of assistive personnel and understanding the philosophy and responsibilities of delegating nursing care.

On some units, registered nurses are cross-trained to do ancillary tasks and function on the principle of "doing it yourself" whenever possible. Other patient-focused areas subscribe to a principle of selecting the right person for the job. Part of the care team is composed of registered nurses working with either unlicensed assistive personnel or certified nursing assistants who are cross-trained.

Another characteristic of this phase of restructuring is the major paradigm shift toward empowering all staff. Patient-focused hospitals provide all levels of employees with the opportunity for increased responsibility and the authority to meet patient needs with established accountability for patient outcomes. Some of the responsibilities that empower staff on patient-focused units include multidisciplinary collaboration and the development and use of practice guidelines, critical paths, and care maps to standardize patient-care processes. The provision of care, which extends across a continuum from an episode of care to an episode of illness, is another characteristic responsibility. Leveraging, a system employed by some patient-focused care hospitals, allows staff to spend an optimal portion of their work time at the high end of their skill level. In other words, staff are empowered to function at a level most consistent with their education and training.

The essence of work redesign is pushing responsibility and authority as far down in the organization as possible. With patient-focused hospitals, the rigid, static structure of the hierarchical pyramid is being replaced by a flatter structure with a very small, well-defined top leadership group. Employees are encouraged to take risks and cross over departmental lines to identify problems and experiment with solutions to them. On many patient-focused care units, teams perform evaluation, supervision, and problem resolution. Decision making is decentralized and requires that staff have responsibility for decisions affecting the cost and quality of care.

While the concepts of process reengineering and work redesign may be implemented separately, many experts believe the best system for organizing work activities features a combination of the two in sequential order. Therefore, this complete restructuring effort of transforming patient care delivery concentrates on the human side of health care, not merely following a set process.

## FROM VISION TO REALITY

No restructuring effort is a low-risk project—especially when an active organization is involved. Work redesign affects the daily work of employees and physicians, a community, and a service area. This necessitates careful review and consideration of all care options. Clearly, the costs—whether measured in direct dollars for consultation, education, training, committee support, and facility modifications, or as indirect costs such as organizational chaos, confusion, resistance, and anger—are high.

Hospitals must realize that patient-focused care transformation requires the involvement of all employees throughout the process. In addition, the commitment of senior management is essential. Without their dedication and support over an extended period of time, change will not occur. Individuals immersed in the restructuring effort will not only better understand the process but also feel a sense of ownership and advocacy that will lead to a successful implementation.

The move to patient care redesign usually proceeds in four phases: vision, design, development, and implementation. A critical first step in beginning the restructuring process is to create the vision. Without an understanding of the plan and goal, the daunting task of restructuring is not possible. The work is too hard, the issues too diverse, and the opportunities for sabotage too easily available.

The creation of a vision must reflect the values of the organization and is the responsibility of senior management. Others usually involved in the process are leaders of the medical staff and members of the project group who will assume responsibility for guiding the vision. The vision must be shared in detail at multiple meetings of hospital medical staff so that all who will become stakeholders in the process can understand the direction of the organization. It is helpful if the chief executive officer of the facility can lead these discussions, thereby reinforcing his or her commitment to the vision and restructuring process.

The vision statement then becomes the foundation for the design phase. Priorities for this stage are determined by the project group. A group of patient care and support department directors creates a project group and is charged with designing a template for inpatient care. For optimum health outcomes, the template can be applied across the entire continuum of care, from pre-hospital to post-discharge care at home.

Staff involvement, which *must* be supported by the organization in both time and dollars, begins during the development phase. This is the phase of customizing the template. Usually one unit is selected as a pilot or demonstration site. To improve the transition to a patient-focused care environment, hospital and unit staff should be involved on all committees that address patient and business aspects of daily activity at the unit level.

The input of staff doing the work is crucial in decision making. Staff input creates a more positive workflow for nurses and creates improved access points to unit support facilities for both staff and patients. New patient care positions may be identified during this phase. Since the positions are new, many organizations give current staff the option of applying for them or being assigned to another position in the organization. Staff who opt not to apply or who are not selected for new roles can be reassigned to remaining traditional units.

A key challenge during the development phase is to carefully plan which services will be deployed to a unit based on that specific patient population. For example, will respiratory care be a factor on this unit? Is the volume of work such that moving the function would make sense? Does the volume of radiography justify the expense of replicating services on a patient-focused unit? Each organization has unique needs in relation to relocating services. Facility modification to implement patient-focused care must be considered and budgeted.

Keep in mind that the transition from traditional delivery system to patient-focused care environment often can be obstructed by a organizational culture that does not want to change, as well as by perceived threats to professional autonomy. It is imperative to rely on communication, leadership, and education to accomplish this goal. During the development phase, it is essential that resource issues involving education, transition of work to the new model, coverage of existing daily work during training, and the readiness of staff to learn and of others to teach are thoroughly assessed. It is not possible to overemphasize the need to attend to all details of these crucial factors.

Enhancing information-sharing and understanding requires a communication strategy. Newsletters, open forums, and meetings must be held for all levels of staff. Support for transitioning staff and options for maintaining employment morale during transition must be discussed and developed. Providing for ongoing opportunities to have open, honest dialogue and allowing for discussion to clarify misconceptions and rumors becomes critical. These communication enhancements will continue to support the implementation process as patient-focused work transformation moves and diffuses to other units.

Although the anxiety and fear created by restructuring an entire organization cannot be eliminated by ongoing quality leadership and communication, these emotions can be successfully managed through quality leadership and the commitment of the facility to transitional education needs. However, developing and maintaining an atmosphere of trust through consistent modeling of desired behaviors across all levels of the organization is essential.

A hospital committee will need to coordinate the education and training components of work redesign. Although the training cycle varies somewhat, the overall process of training usually occurs over a 12-week period. "Team training" is a major element of the education plan, and addresses the complex issue of how individuals on the teams will work together on a daily basis in a restructured system.

Clearly, significant resources need to be committed to the didactic education portion of patient-focused redesign; however, it is equally important that there be resources to support implementation of the model. Patient-focused work transformation is a *process*, not a "light switch" operation. Ongoing support of all staff is a critical success factor. Both staff's support of the process and administrative support of the staff are mandatory for success. Whether registered nursing staff are addressing delegation and conflict resolution or non-professional staff are accepting the challenges of cross-training, the work group as an entity is new. Often, the numbers of staff involved are large and the dynamics of work groups, tasks, and skills will remain a challenge for an extended period of time.

It is *unrealistic and an invitation to failure* to assume an organization can be restructured without significant resources invested in training. As Mitchell Lee Marks states in his book *From Turmoil to Triumph* (1994), people change in two ways: either by design or by default. An organization will have employees defaulting to their own unique ways of doing things unless a specifically designed organizational transition strategy is created by the senior leadership.

Indeed, excellent leadership skills are an essential factor for the success of any project. The leader certainly must have vision for what the model will become, and passion for the concepts of patient-focused care. He or she should be a strong, empowered communicator and empathetic listener. In addition, being mature, clinically sound, respected, and committed to the model and staff are crucial leadership characteristics.

To overcome potential cultural barriers to change, such as fear of the unknown and high costs/low returns, lack of clarity and trust, too little involvement, and loss of job security, skilled management is required. Certainly, for optimal results, there must be strong and visible leadership, a frequent and interactive presence on the part of senior management, and face-to-face support from consultants or internal management development staff, educators, and others who can "walk the talk" of change.

Reviewing the intricacies of complex change theory with those involved in providing the support, as well as with the staff experiencing the transformation, is extremely important. All involved, including senior management, unit leadership, and clinical staff, need to relearn sophisticated current change and chaos theory to know what "normal" is and where they fit in the new model. Trust and team-building take time—and they are built on small successes. Remember, support for even the smallest accomplishments needs to be provided.

Keep in mind, too, that learning curves will vary depending on the baseline knowledge and skills of those assigned to the unit as well as on the quality of the leadership available. Importantly, support must be committed to assist leaders and staff on a daily basis, since the requisite skills on the transformed unit require successful application and ongoing practice. Failure to attend to this key element will diminish an otherwise successful transformation.

The final phase of demonstration also includes ongoing improvement. Although it is the "last" phase, nothing is ever complete. Refinements continue to be made as patient-focused work transformation diffuses to other units. The specific implementation strategies will vary from unit to unit, while the basic restricting concepts remain consistently applied.

Staff will continue to benefit from the initial efforts of the original start-up unit, and modify their plans according to assessments of what worked and what did not. Decisions and adjustments must be data-driven, not intuitive.

Additionally, it is vital that staff perceive that they are supported as they make this transition and that problem-solving is ongoing and facilitated. To reinforce the complexity of the project and to ensure that seemingly simple pieces of the patient-focused puzzle do not threaten to affect successful implementation, leaders must commit to the model and show visible support to staff. Management also must keep in mind that more staff are needed on a temporary basis during demonstration and for support of the education process.

Leaders also need to remember that new roles will require clarification and reinforcement over and over again. To this end, daily team planning meetings on units are essential. When they do not occur, work does not become well orchestrated. Likewise, clinical competency reviews for all staff need to be ongoing, and close communication between central departments and the transitional units must occur. Moreover, physicians should be involved at every possible juncture to increase opportunities for collaboration.

As with any project, measurement indicators must be identified and must be shared with all stakeholders. Without known indicators, neither staff nor management will realize whether success has been achieved. The indicators that are usually identified for continuous measurement are patient, staff, and physician satisfaction; clinical outcomes; and financial performance. Begin collecting the data at the "go live" date of the demonstration unit. Depending on the facility, some elements are measured daily while others are collected weekly, monthly, or quarterly. Data are normally reviewed formally on a monthly basis. Evaluation of data usually includes achievement of clinical outcomes; any change in length of stay; and patient, staff, and physician satisfaction. It is not unusual to have the physician satisfaction with the model rise and fall depending on staff satisfaction. Staff satisfaction tends to reflect the delivery system's newness and their own evolving skills; both continue to improve over time.

An organization's senior management team must recognize the long-term benefit of patient-focused work transformation and that the organization will still be involved with the expenses of supporting multiple or dual systems (traditional and patient-focused work transformation) during the transition. Therefore, full cost savings are not yet realized at the time of implementation. It is probably unreasonable for facilities to predict or expect cost savings of greater than 10 percent in operations over a two-to-three-year period. It often takes almost a full year to have all inpatient areas functioning as patient-focused work transformation units. Despite the ongoing and continuous challenges, hospitals need to remain committed to creating a patient-focused delivery system. Staff must feel that the vision is solid and the plan will work.

The issue of restructuring health care organizations requires making hard decisions about how to best meet the needs of patients while containing cost. To achieve success, hospitals—first and foremost—need a vision. Like any other corporation, their strategies must be directed to provide marketable, quality service at a reasonable cost. Patient-focused care provides that opportunity.

The nursing community must also be prepared and willing to create a vision that is inclusive rather than exclusive. They must commit to participate fully in the intense process of change. Those for whom control continues to be an issue of both style and substance had best update their resumes. The restructuring organization will demand only your best and most creative efforts. Staff will and should be able to expect that commitment of the organization and leadership will be complete.

Patient-focused work transformation is a formidable task. No one organization has all the answers, but the reality is that change is linear and never ceases. Take time to look outside yourself and anticipate change. Then, change *before* you have to. By doing so you will have created the future, not simply reacted to it!

## DISCUSSION QUESTIONS

1. Is patient-focused care a reengineering strategy? Why or why not?
2. Has reengineering been done by health care providers in your geographic area? Has it been successful? Why or why not?

3. List five benefits and five disadvantages to reengineering a health care facility. Discuss.

4. What would make reengineering a successful undertaking, if it has been unsuccessfully attempted thus far, for nurses in your geographic location? Why?

---

**BIBLIOGRAPHY**

American Association of Critical-Care Nurses. 1996. "Decision Grid for Delegation." Staffing Tool Kit. Aliso Viejo, California: AACN Publishing.

American Nurses' Association. 1993. *Nursing's Agenda for Health Care Reform.* Washington, D.C.: ANA Publishing.

———. 1994. *Every Patient Deserves a Nurse.* Brochure. Washington, D.C.: ANA Publishing.

———. 1996. *Registered Professional Nurses and Unlicensed Assistive Personnel.* 2nd ed. Washington, D.C.: ANA Publishing.

American Organization of Nurse Executives. 1996. *Talking Points on Hospital Redesign.* Washington, D.C.: American Organization of Nurse Executives.

Ashton, J., and Fike, R., eds. 1996. *Reengineering for Patient-Focused Care.* Boston: Prescott Publishing.

Beckham, J.D. 1997a. "The Right Way to Integrate." *Healthcare Forum Journal,* July/ August, 30–37.

———. 1997b. "The Beginning of the End for HMOs." Part 1. *Healthcare Forum Journal,* November/December, 44–47.

———. 1998. "The Beginning of the End for HMOs." Part 2. *Healthcare Forum Journal,* January/February, 52–55.

Bergman, R. 1994. "Reengineering Health Care." *Hospitals and Health Networks,* 5 February, 16–24.

Beyers, M. 1996. "The Value of Nursing." *Hospitals and Health Networks,* 5 February, 52.

Bridges, W. 1980. *Transitions.* Boston: Addison Wesley Publishing.

———. 1988. *Surviving Corporate Transition.* New York: Doubleday.

Brink, S. et al. 1997. "America's Top HMOs." *US News and World Report,* 13 October, 60–69.

Burda, D. 1994a. "A Profit by Any Other Name Would Still Give Hospitals the Fits." *Modern Healthcare,* 8 August, 115–136.

———. 1994b. "Layoffs Rise as Pace of Cost-Cutting Accelerates." *Modern Healthcare,* 12 December, 32.

———. 1995. "ANA Report Stokes Restructuring Debate." *Modern Healthcare,* 13 February, 38.

Burns, J. 1993. "Caring for the Community." *Modern Healthcare*, 8 November, 30–33.

Butts, J., and Brock, A. 1996. "Optimizing Nursing through Reorganization: Mandates for the New Millennium." *Nursing Connections* 9(4): 5–10.

Byrne, J. 1993. "The Horizontal Corporation." *Business Week*, 20 December, 76–81.

California Nurses Association. Web Site Home Page. http://www.califnurses.org/

California Taxpayers Against Higher Health Costs. 1996. Ballot materials.

Chriss, L. 1996. "Nurses Learn How to Work with Assistants." *NurseWeek*, 30 September, 1–3.

Christensen, P., and Bender, L. 1994. "Models of Nursing Care in a Changing Environment." *Orthopaedic Nursing* 13(2): 64–70.

Clarkson Hospital. 1995. "Patient Focused Care." Presentation handouts, June 1995, Omaha, Nebraska.

Coile, R. 1993a. "California Healthcare 2001: The Outlook for America's Bellwether State." *Hospital Strategy Report* 5(4), February.

———. 1993b. "California Hospitals in the 21st Century." *California Hospitals*, November/December, 7–10.

———. 1994a. "Primary Care Networks: The Integrators of Care in an Integrated Delivery System." *Hospital Strategy Report* 6(8): 1–3.

———. 1994b. "Capitation: The New Food Chain of HMO Provider Payment." *Hospital Strategy Report* 6(9): 1–3.

Curran, C., ed. 1990. "IDN Core Competencies and Nursing's Role." *Nursing Economics*, December.

Davis, C., ed. 1996. *Nursing Staff in Hospitals and Nursing Homes: Is It Adequate?* National Institute of Medicine. Baltimore: National Academy Press.

Donaho, B., ed. 1996. *Celebrating the Journey: A Final Report on Strengthening Hospital Nursing*. Philadelphia: National Academy Press.

Dracup, K., and Bryan-Brown, C., eds. 1998. "Thinking Outside the Box and Other Resolutions." *American Journal of Critical-Care*, January, 1.

Eck, S. et al. 1997. "Consumerism, Nursing and the Reality of Resources." *Nursing Administration Quarterly* 12(3): 1–11.

Flower, J. 1997a. "Job Shift." *Healthcare Forum Journal*, January/February, 15–24.

Flower, J. 1997b. "The Age of Heretics." *Healthcare Forum Journal*, March/April, 34–39.

Fralicx, R., and Bolster, C.J. 1997. "Preventing Culture Shock." *Modern Healthcare*, 11 August, 50.

Goldsmith, J. 1993. "Driving the Nitroglycerin Truck," *Healthcare Forum Journal*, March/April, 36–44.

———. 1996. "Managed Care Mythology: Supply Dreams Die Hard." *Healthcare Forum Journal*, November/December, 43–47.

Golub, E. 1995. "Revisiting Our Ideas About Health." *Hospitals and Health Networks*, 20 January, 78.

Goodman, J. 1993. "Twenty Myths About National Health Insurance." National Center for Policy Analysis, Dallas, Texas.

Goss, T. et al. 1993. "Risking the Present for a Powerful Future." *Harvard Business Review*, November/December, 98–108.

Gray, B.B. 1994a. "Twenty-First Century Hospital Embodies New Concept." *NurseWeek*, 1 April, 1.

———. 1994b. "Changing Skill Mix Reorders Healthcare Delivery System." *NurseWeek*, 2 December, 14.

———. 1995. "Issues at the Crossroads." Parts 1 and 2. *NurseWeek*, 1 October, 1.

Hall, G. et al. 1993. "How to Make Reengineering Really Work." *Harvard Business Review*, November/December, 119–131.

Hammer, M., and Champy, J. 1993. *Reengineering the Corporation*. New York: Harper Business.

Hammers, M.A. 1994. "Crystal Ball Gazing with Leland Kaiser." *RN Times*, 5 September, 8–10.

Harrington, C., and Estes, C., eds. 1997. *Health Policy and Nursing*. 2nd ed. Boston: Jones and Barlett.

Healthcare Advisory Board. 1992a. "Executive Report to the CEO: The Merits of Patient-Focused Care." Acetate presentation, October, The Advisory Board Company, Washington, D.C.

———. 1992b. "Toward a Twenty-First Century Hospital: Designing Patient Care." Acetate presentation, October, The Advisory Board Company, Washington, D.C.

Heifetz, M. 1993. *Leading Change, Overcoming Chaos*. Berkeley, CA: Ten Speed Press.

Hirsch, G. 1997. "Fit to Be Tried." *Hospitals and Health Networks*, 5 November, 50–54.

Izzo, J. 1998. "The Changing Values of Workers." *Healthcare Forum Journal*, May/June, 62–65.

Jaffe, D., and Scott, C. 1997. "The Human Side of Reengineering." *Healthcare Forum Journal*, September/October, 14–21.

Kanter, R.M. 1983. *The Change Masters*. New York: Simon and Schuster.

Katzenbaach, J.R., and Smith, D.K. 1993. *The Wisdom of Teams*. New York: Harper Collins.

Keepnews, D., and Marullo, G. 1996. "Policy Imperatives for Nursing in an Era of Healthcare Restructuring." *Nursing Administration Quarterly* 20(3): 19–31 (spring).

Kertesz, L. 1997. "What's Right, Wrong?" *Modern Healthcare*, 11 August, 70–74.

Kunen, J. 1996. "The New Hands-Off Nursing." *Time*, 30 September, 55–57.

Lanara, V.A. 1993. "The Nurse of the Future, Role and Function." *Journal of Nursing Management* 1: 83–87.

Larson, C.E., and LaFasto, F.M. 1989. *Teamwork: What Must Go Right, What Can Go Wrong*. Newbury Park, California: Sage Publications.

Lumsdon, K. 1994a. "It's a Jungle Out There!" *Hospitals and Health Networks*, 20 May, 68–72.

———. 1994b. "Want to Save Millions?" *Hospitals and Health Networks*, 5 November, 24–32.

———. 1995a. "Working Smarter, Not Harder." *Hospitals and Health Networks*, 5 November, 27–31.

———. 1995b. "Faded Glory." *Hospitals and Health Networks*, 5 December, 31–36.

MacStravic, S. 1988. "Outcome Marketing in Healthcare." *Healthcare Management Review* 13(2): 53–59.

———. 1997. "Managing Demand: The Wrong Paradigm." *Managed Care Quarterly* 5(4): 8–17.

Malone, B. et al. 1996. "A Grim Prognosis for Healthcare." *American Journal of Nursing Survey Results*, November, 40.

Manthey, M. 1994. "Issues in Patient Care Delivery." *Journal of Nursing Administration* 24(12): 14–16.

Manuel, P., and Sorensen, L. 1995. "Changing Trends in Healthcare: Implications for Baccalaureate Education, Practice and Employment." *Journal of Nursing Education* 34(6): 248–53.

Marks, M. 1994. *From Turmoil to Triumph*. New York: Lexington Press.

Martin, R. 1993. "Changing the Mind of the Corporation." *Harvard Business Review*, November/December, 81–94.

Mauer, R. 1996. *Beyond the Wall of Resistance*. Austin, Texas: Bard Books, Inc.

McCloskey, J., and Grace, H. 1997. *Current Issues in Nursing*. 5th ed. New York: Mosby.

McManis, G.L. 1993. "Reinventing the System." *Hospitals and Health Networks*, 5 October, 42–48.

Merisalo, L., ed. 1998. "RN Staff Cuts Due to Managed Care Pressures May Be Costly." *Managed Care Payment Advisor*, March, 1–2.

Miller, J. 1995. "Leading Nursing into the Future." *Harvard Nursing Research Institute Newsletter* 4(3): 5–7 (summer).

Moore, J.D., Jr. 1998. "What Downsizing." *Modern Healthcare*, 19 January, 12.

Morrell, J. 1995. "Turn Your Focus Outside In." *Hospitals and Health Networks*, 5 December, 66.

National Council of Nursing State Boards. 1995. "Delegation." *Issues 95* 15(1): 1–3.

Olmos, D. 1997. "HMO Panel to Call for Consumer Protections." *Los Angeles Times*, 31 December, 1.

Organization of Nurse Leaders. 1995. Focus Group Notes. *Nursing Issues*. 29 September.

O'Rourke, M.W. 1996. "Who Holds the Keys to the Future of Healthcare?" *NurseWeek*, 8 January, 1.

Pallarito, K. 1996. "Deloitte Survey Identifies Service Consolidation as Key to Efficiency." *Modern Healthcare*, 24 June, 3.

Pew Health Professions Commission. 1995. "Healthy America: Practitioners for 2005." *Pew Health Professions Report*. Washington, D.C.: Pew Health Professions Commission.

————. 1998. " *Pew Health Professions Report*. Washington, D.C.: Pew Health Professions Commission.

Pinto, C. et al. 1998. "Future Trends." *Modern Healthcare*, 5 January, 27–40.

Porter-O'Grady, T. 1994. "Working with Consultants on a Redesign." *American Journal of Nursing,* October, 33–39.

Prokesch, S. 1993. "Mastering Chaos at the High-Tech Frontier." *Harvard Business Review*, November/December, 135–144.

Public Policy Institute of California. 1996. *Nursing Staff Trends in California Hospitals: 1977–1995.* October. Sacramento, California: Public Policy Institute of California.

Rich, P.L. 1995. "Working with Nursing Assistants: Becoming a Team." *Nursing 95*, May, 100–103.

RN Scope of Practice, California Business and Professions Code, sec. 2725.

RN Special Advisory Committee. 1990. *Meeting the Immediate and Future Needs for Nursing in California.* Sacramento, California: State of California.

Sheehy, B. et al. 1995. "Don't Blink or You'll Miss It." *The Atlanta Consulting Group*, Atlanta, 69–87.

Shelton, K., ed. 1995. *Executive Excellence Magazine*, February.

Sherer, J. 1994a. "Corporate Cultures." *Hospitals and Health Networks*, 5 May, 20–27.

————. 1994b. "Job Shifts." *Hospitals and Health Networks*, 5 October, 64–68.

————. 1994c. "Union Uprising: California Nurses React Aggressively to Work Redesign." *Hospitals and Health Networks*, 20 December, 36–38.

————. 1995. "Tapping into Teams." *Hospitals and Health Networks*, 5 July, 32–35.

Shindul-Rothschild, J. et al. 1997. "Ten Keys to Quality Care." *American Journal of Nursing* 97(11): 35–43.

Shortell, S. et al. 1996. *Remaking Healthcare in America*. San Francisco: Jossey-Bass.

Shubert, D. 1996. "Hospitals Decrease Nurses' Role: Reassign Tasks to Aides." *Los Angeles Times*, 14 July.

Simmons, H. 1998. "The Forces That Impact Healthcare-Quality and Costs." *Healthcare Forum Journal*, January/February, 27–46.

Stewart, T. 1993. "Reengineering: The Hot New Management Tool." *Fortune*, 23 August, 41–45.

St. Vincent Hospital. 1994. "CARE 2000: An Approach to Patient Focused Care." Presentation handouts, February 1994.

Teisberg, E. et al. 1994. "Making Competition in Health Care Work." *Harvard Business Review*, July/August, 131–141.

Truscott, J.P., and Churchill, G.M. 1995. "Patient Focused Care." *Nursing Policy Forum* 1(4): 5–12.

Turner, S.O. 1995a. "Laid Off: Now What?" *Nursing 95*, May, 94–95.

————. 1995b. "Reality Check: It's Time for Nursing to Face the Future." *Hospitals and Health Networks*, 20 August, 20–22.

———. 1995c. "Nurses: Are They the Key to Successful Capitation?" *Capitation and Medical Practice*, December, 1–2.

———. 1996. "Capitation: Are You Ready for It?" *Surgical Services Management*, February, 43–45.

Udvarhelyi, I.S. et al. 1994. "Perspectives: Finding a Lasting Cure for US Healthcare." *Harvard Business Review*, September/October, 45–63.

Ummel, S. 1997. "Integration." *Healthcare Forum Journal*, March/April, 13–27.

Van, S. 1994. "A New Attitude." *RN Times*, November, 12–13.

Weissenstein, E., and Pallarito, K. 1994. "Senate Plan Adds to Reform Confusion." *Modern Healthcare*, 8 August, 2.

Wesorick, B. "Standards: On the Cutting Edge or Over the Cliff?" *Notes on Clinical Practice, 1990s*. Unpublished paper.

# CHAPTER 8

# Change: The New Constant

Change is paradigm-free thinking, according to some, but it is also a disruptive presence in health care. Never have the effects of change been so widespread, intense, and unceasing as they are today. As William Bridges says in his book *Surviving Corporate Transition*, "change would be easier to manage if we knew where it was headed" (Bridges, 1988, p. 7) Bridges believes that change occurs when something new starts or something old stops. It takes place in a particular point in time.

Change is explained by early twentieth century psychologist Kurt Lewin as a three-step process. First is the unfreezing phase, which is assessment of current culture and environment followed by culture shock and transition. The second phase is the actual changing, where new behaviors are exhibited. The third and final phase is refreezing. The behaviors become new culture (Margulies and Raia, 1972). There are simultaneous pushing and resisting forces for and against change, competing for energy within the organization. When evaluating the pushing and resisting forces, the preferred strategy for dealing with organizational change is to reduce the resisting forces rather than increase the pushing forces. Dealing with change causes conflict, and conflict in organizations causes stress. Changes cause stress, even though positive outcomes occur and much learning takes place.

Change is managed through organizational development. Health care entities, including hospitals, focus on clinical education and training rather than organizational development. Organizational development is defined as the system-wide application of behavioral science knowledge to the planned development and reinforcement of organizational strategies, structures, and processes for improving an organization's effectiveness (Hitt et al., 1986).

Bridges believes that the frequency of change is fed by technology, the accelerated pace of product development, increased competition, and increased expectations of quality. He also notes: "The people trauma in the whole change process almost guarantees that there won't be a productivity increase for a considerable period of time . . . . they're scared to death" (p. 34).

That has certainly been the case in much of the health care industry. Organizational change in health care has resulted from new technology and knowledge, and the impact on the social and economic environment through consumer demands. Resource availability and social attitudes also have determined the pace of change. Health care issues are now financial and social policy issues and this reality fuels the rate of change in health care.

There are several stages of the change process that occur in organizational change. The first is Stage 1. This stage includes shock and fear, an "Oh my God!" reaction. Stage 2 consists of defensive retreat. This phase may include obstructionist behavior and defensive militant responses to new organizational policies and systems. Stage 3 is the acknowledgment that change needs to occur. It includes employees accepting the necessity of change and the need to participate in the process. They recognize the organization's need to change in order to survive, and they become involved in actual redesign of work. The final stage, Stage 4, consists of adaptation and change occurring within the organization (Hitt et al., 1986).

The job of managers is to educate, support, communicate with, and involve employees in change. Staff as well as management may transition through a grieving process as they move from old ways to new. Management needs to recognize this process and prepare for it.

The responsibilities of employees during change are critical. The job of staff is to help themselves and each other deal with change by becoming educated about the changes taking place and the rationale for those changes. Communication with each other and management keeps confu-

Many employees can resist change. Resistance to change is caused by many factors, some of which include:

- employee attitudes and work habits
- anxiety
- organizational cohesiveness
- lack of trust; questioning the motives of others
- too much confidence in the past
- job security and entitlement issues
- uninformed about national changes in health care
- tunnel vision

It is normal for change to cause conflict, fear, and confusion, and to give rise to an urge to return to the "old ways." To question the familiar may take more courage than investigating the unfamiliar.

sion to a minimum and facilitates mutual trust. Staff need to participate in and support changes by facilitating and influencing the change process. This may include negotiating conflicts to achieve resolution. Many health care professionals have debated who is responsible for becoming informed—employees or employers. While teams and groups are the building blocks of organizations, individuals make up teams and groups. Individuals are accountable for understanding change as it will affect their individual performance. They are also responsible for supporting change to enhance the overall success of the organization as well as outlining areas of concern for further review and discussion with management and employees together.

Successful organizations foster collaborative, not competitive, environments, avoiding turf protection and power plays for employees and managers. Effective teams participate with management in decision making around applicable and available resources. This has not always been the case in the health care environment. Many changes, especially in hospitals, have been made by administrators and non-clinical staff—those without hands-on knowledge of the effects of the proposed changes.

Organizational goals should be outlined in an organization's strategic plan. This plan should direct individuals and groups in managing their work amid changing systems. Individuals and interdisciplinary groups must participate in planning and implementing change; they will support what they help create, including redesign of work.

Managing change begins with assessing the existing culture and environment, then creating a new process and plan. Effective communication skills are vital during change. Don't underestimate the value of "over-communicating." During change, it is important to keep everyone in the feedback loop. In addition, conflict management skills are necessary during change. Conflict develops when different values collide, and it is important to manage conflict to resolution instead of burying it. Rick Mauer, in his book *Beyond the Wall of Resistance* (1995), writes that resistance kills change. He states that ideas fail not on their individual merit, but on inability to handle staff resistance. Lack of user involvement is the single largest reason for failure in organizations. The human toll of failure is decreased trust and increased blame of management. These perceptions make further change more difficult.

Mauer believes that managers can work with resistance instead of against it to increase success and decrease the time it takes to implement change. He believes that resisters deserve respect and that keeping relationships with resisters intact builds stronger relationships and provides a solid base for the success of future change (1995).

## DEALING WITH CHANGE AT WORK

This section could also be called "Dealing with Managed Care." Most of the health care changes discussed in this book are about managed care. While you may not like what is happening, recognizing and coping with it will make your nursing career successful.

Coping with change and transition at work begins with believing in it. Accept that managed health care is happening and understand that you cannot always control the changes it has brought with it. Attempts to obstruct change can result in you being perceived as a difficult employee— which puts you at the front of the line during layoffs and downsizing. It also makes managers think twice before asking for your assistance or rewarding your efforts.

You can't afford to lose your credibility and integrity. Militancy is not the answer; it just makes you look obstructive. Managed care is not going to go away. It may be tweaked and continue to be redefined, but it is here to stay. Unless you plan to retire or leave the nursing profession, chances are you will need to learn to deal with a managed care environment.

To be successful in the present marketplace, you must be perceived as a valuable employee. Employers have specific ideas about what constitutes a valuable employee. There are certain competencies and characteristics in nurses that make them invaluable to the organization.

Nurses need to be clinically competent in more than one area or specialty. The specialty areas can be related to each other, such as postpartum and labor and delivery or surgery and post-anesthesia recovery. It is important to be perceived as flexible within your clinical skills inventory.

Nurses need to have a general understanding of the standards and criteria of the Joint Commission on Accreditation of Healthcare Organizations, as well as state regulations. In addition, general understanding of the Nurse Practice Act, scope of practice, and standards of competent performance is needed. Your awareness of managed care concepts, budgeting, cost, and reimbursement issues is helpful to employers who need to be reassured that nursing employees understand what hospitals and health care facilities are facing.

To be perceived as valuable, nurses need to demonstrate a willingness to partner with the institution, to be more than just an employee. Instead of the "us versus them" mentality, these nurses demonstrate the "us helping them" mentality. The nurses held in highest esteem by employers are those who are seen as "in it knee-deep with everyone else."

Certain personality characteristics go with the skills competencies discussed above. Nurses considered valuable employees demonstrate decision-making skills used with self-direction. These nurses have a high level of energy and a strong work ethic but are not workaholics. They demonstrate an objective perspective as an independent thinker, not as a victim to the organizational changes going on in their institutions. They act with integrity and honesty. They are self-motivated, demonstrate personal initiative, and continually show a willingness to learn.

An organization's most valued employees demonstrate effective time management skills and can be counted on routinely to cope well with situations that other nurses believe to be difficult or impossible. These staff members show a strong and positive self-image. They are assertive but not aggressive, and consistently demonstrate tenacity and personal ambition.

In addition, they are enthusiastic about—not threatened by—change. Keep in mind that fear of change is normal, but immobilization is not. Nurses who can demonstrate adaptability after dealing with the fear and uncertainty of change are highly prized. They demonstrate the most important characteristic of all—flexibility.

One personality characteristic of nurses most valued by their employers is the ability to cope with ambiguity. Coping with ambiguity in this setting means being comfortable with one foot in the past and the other in the future. Another characteristic appreciated by employers is the ability to manage oneself through a transition and not act like a victim.

Prized nurses have consistently effectual interpersonal skills. They are able to communicate their institution's vision and mission clearly to other employees and patients, as well as demonstrate those concepts in their caregiving.

These individuals provide positive professional role modeling for other employees. They trust their colleagues and other health care professionals, and, in turn, foster trust in others. They show strong problem-solving and decision-making skills, as well as consistently demonstrating the critical-thinking process while solving problems.

In addition, these staff members maintain a reasonable perspective of the environment they work in and those around them. They usually don't become emotional and reactive to difficult situations. They maintain and use a sense of humor with colleagues and co-workers. They work well in teams and have the ability to influence others. These nurses value caregivers as resources and are able to foster innovation in others they work with or supervise.

Such individuals act as change agents. They become a spark for other employees to respond to change proactively. They actively pursue self-development, including job- and career-enhancing strategies such as cross-training, obtaining a BSN, or learning new transition skills.

These employees realize that there are certain tasks, policies, and situations that staff or organizations may not be able to address—and accept this. They do not perceive themselves as personally ineffective when they are unable to create a change in their work environment.

Valuable nurse employees seek management support to deal with issues and encourage others to do the same. They do not whine about how things *used* to be but rather verbalize how things *could* be. These nurses are truly valuable to their organization and will both accept the risks and achieve the rewards of adding value to their workplace.

In reality, there are both risks and rewards of adding value and being perceived as valuable to the workplace. The risks include the inability to be positive all the time, increased stress, lack of job security, and dealing with ambiguity consistently.

Nurses who embrace change also may be seen as traitors by colleagues for "siding with management" and may feel "caught in the middle" frequently when issues arise or incidents occur. These staff have to guard against a continual crisis-oriented mentality, but realize "business as usual" is no longer effective.

They will experience the risk and actuality of failure as well as changing peer and management relationships and isolation from other staff members as an organizational "odd duck."

The rewards of being perceived as valuable in your workplace include continued employment as well as empowerment. You will experience increased self-confidence, achieve personal growth, and have many opportunities to be innovative and creative. You can generate pride and professionalism in your nursing work. This will lead to expanding horizons and job options.

## DISCUSSION QUESTIONS

1. Have change and transition been well managed by health care providers in your geographic location? Why or why not?
2. Have change and transition been well managed by nurses in your geographic location? Why or why not?
3. List five strategies for managing change and transition that would be likely to be successful in your geographic area.
4. Identify and describe any behaviors you have seen demonstrated by nurses in your geographic area that would indicate whether change has been accepted or not. Explain your interpretation of the behaviors identified.
5. How do most of your professional nursing colleagues deal with change at work? Are they successful? Why or why not?
6. Identify six strategies for coping proactively with change in the workplace.

**BIBLIOGRAPHY**

Adizes, S. 1993. *Mastering Change.* Pacific Palisades, California: Adizes Institute Publications.

Aiken, L. et al. 1994. "Lower Medicare Mortality among a Set of Hospitals Known for Good Nursing Care." *Medical Care* 32(8): 771–785.

Ashton, J., and Fike, R., eds. 1996. *Reengineering for Patient-Focused Care.* Boston: Prescott Publishing.

Bayley, E. et al. 1997. "Preparing to Change from Acute to Community Based Care." *Journal of Nursing Administration* 27:5.

Beckham, J.D. 1997. "The Right Way to Integrate." *Healthcare Forum Journal,* July/August, 30–37.

Bergman, R. 1993. "Quantum Leaps." *Hospitals and Health Networks,* 5 October, 28–35.

———. 1994. "Reengineering Health Care." *Hospitals and Health Networks,* 5 February, 16–24.

Bernard, L., and Walsh, M. 1996. *Leadership: The Key to Professionalization of Nursing.* New York: Mosby.

Beyers, M. 1996. "The Value of Nursing." *Hospitals and Health Networks,* 5 February, 52.

Bolen, D., and Unland, J. 1994. "Surviving Stress." *Hospitals and Health Networks,* 20 October, 100.

Bridges, W. 1980. *Transitions.* Boston: Addison Wesley Publishing.

———. 1988. *Surviving Corporate Transition.* New York: Doubleday.

Brink, S. et al. 1997. "America's Top HMOs." *US News and World Report,* 13 October, 60–69.

Brock, R. 1996. "Head for Business." *Hospitals and Health Networks,* 5 December, 62–66.

Burda, D. 1994. "A Profit by Any Other Name Would Still Give Hospitals the Fits." *Modern Healthcare,* 8 August, 115–136.

———. 1995. "ANA Report Stokes Restructuring Debate." *Modern Healthcare,* 13 February, 38.

Burns, J. 1993. "Caring for the Community." *Modern Healthcare,* 8 November, 30–33.

Butts, J., and Brock, A. 1996. "Optimizing Nursing through Reorganization: Mandates for the New Millennium." *Nursing Connections* 9(4): 5–10.

Byrne, J. 1993. "The Horizontal Corporation." *Business Week,* 20 December, 76–81.

California Strategic Planning Committee for Nursing. 1996. *Final Report.* Irvine, California: California Strategic Planning Committee for Nursing.

Chriss, L. 1996. "Nurses Learn How to Work with Assistants." *NurseWeek,* 30 September, 1–3.

Christensen, P., and Bender, L. 1994. "Models of Nursing Care in a Changing Environment." *Orthopaedic Nursing* 13(2): 64–70.

Clarkson Hospital. 1995. "Patient Focused Care." Presentation handouts, June 1995, Omaha, Nebraska.

Coile, R. 1993a. "California Healthcare 2001: The Outlook for America's Bellwether State." *Hospital Strategy Report* 5(4), February.

———. 1993b. "California Hospitals in the 21st Century." *California Hospitals*, November/December, 7–10.

———. 1994a. "Primary Care Networks: The Integrators of Care in an Integrated Delivery System." *Hospital Strategy Report* 6(8): 1–3.

———. 1994b. "Capitation: The New Food Chain of HMO Provider Payment." *Hospital Strategy Report* 6(9): 1–3.

Collins, H.L. 1989. "How Well Do Nurses Nurture Themselves?" *RN*, May, 39–41.

Commonwealth Fund. 1995. *Healthcare Statistics*. Washington, D.C.: US Health Care Financing Administration.

Conti, R. 1996. "Nurse Case Manager Roles: Implications for Practice." *Nursing Administration Quarterly* 21:1.

Curran, C., ed. 1990. "IDN Core Competencies and Nursing's Role." *Nursing Economics*, December.

Davis, C., ed. 1996. *Nursing Staff in Hospitals and Nursing Homes: Is It Adequate?* National Institute of Medicine. Baltimore: National Academy Press.

Donaho, B., ed. 1996. *Celebrating the Journey: A Final Report on Strengthening Hospital Nursing*. Philadelphia: National Academy Press.

Dracup, K., and Bryan-Brown, C., eds. 1998. "Thinking Outside the Box and Other Resolutions." *American Journal of Critical-Care*, January, 1.

Duck, J.D. 1993. "Managing Change: The Art of Balancing." *Harvard Business Review*, November/December, 109–118.

Federwisch, A. 1997. "Teammates or Adversaries? Your Attitude Matters." *NurseWeek*, 13 October, 1.

———. 1998. "Attitude Matters." *NurseWeek*, 26 January, 13.

Flower, J. 1997a. "Job Shift." *Healthcare Forum Journal*, January/February, 15–24.

———. 1997b. "The Age of Heretics." *Healthcare Forum Journal*, March/April, 34–39.

Fralicx, R., and Bolster, C.J. 1997. "Preventing Culture Shock." *Modern Healthcare*, 11 August, 50.

Gray, B.B. 1994a. "Twenty-First Century Hospital Embodies New Concept." *NurseWeek*, 1 April, 1.

———. 1994b. "Changing Skill Mix Reorders Healthcare Delivery System." *NurseWeek*, 2 December, 14.

———. 1995a. "Nurses Face Ethics of Rationing as Healthcare Industry Evolves." *NurseWeek*, 2 April, 20–22.

———. 1995b. "Issues at the Crossroads." Parts 1 and 2. *NurseWeek*, 1 October, 1.

Grayson, M., ed. 1997. "Stuck on a Strategy." *Hospitals and Health Networks*, 5 October, 74–76.

Hall, G. et al. 1993. "How to Make Reengineering Really Work." *Harvard Business Review*, November/December, 119–31.

Hammer, M., and Champy, J. 1995. *Reengineering the Corporation*. New York: Harper Business.

Hammers, M.A. 1994. "Crystal Ball Gazing with Leland Kaiser." *RN Times*, 5 September, 8–10.

Harrington, C., and Estes, C., eds. 1997. *Health Policy and Nursing*. 2nd ed. Boston: Jones and Barlett.

Heifetz, M. 1993. *Leading Change, Overcoming Chaos*. Berkeley, CA: Ten Speed Press.

Hirsch, G. 1997. "Fit to Be Tried." *Hospitals and Health Networks*, 5 November, 50–54.

Hitt, M., Middlemist, R., and Mathis, R. 1986. *Management Concepts and Effective Practice*. 2nd ed. Houston, Texas: West Publishing.

Izzo, J. 1998. "The Changing Values of Workers." *Healthcare Forum Journal*, May/June, 62–65.

Jaffe, D., and Scott, C. 1997. "The Human Side of Reengineering." *Healthcare Forum Journal*, September/October, 14–21.

Kanter, R.M. 1983. *The Change Masters*. New York: Simon and Schuster.

―――. 1990. *When Giants Learn to Dance*. New York: Simon and Schuster.

Katzenbaach, J.R., and Smith, D.K. 1993. *The Wisdom of Teams*. New York: Harper Collins.

Kemp, V.H. 1995. "Overview of Change and Leadership." *Contemporary Leadership Behavior*. 2nd ed. Boston: Little Brown and Company.

Kertesz, L. 1997. "What's Right, Wrong?" *Modern Healthcare*, 11 August, 70–74.

Kunen, J. 1996. "The New Hands-Off Nursing." *Time*, 30 September, 55–57.

Lanara, V.A. 1993. "The Nurse of the Future, Role and Function." *Journal of Nursing Management* 1: 83–87.

Larson, C.E., and LaFasto, F.M. 1989. *Teamwork: What Must Go Right, What Can Go Wrong*. Newbury Park, California: Sage Publications.

Lumsdon, K. 1995a. "Working Smarter, Not Harder." *Hospitals and Health Networks*, 5 November, 27–31.

―――. 1995b. "Faded Glory." *Hospitals and Health Networks*, 5 December, 31–36.

MacStravic, S. 1997. "Managing Demand: The Wrong Paradigm." *Managed Care Quarterly* 5(4): 8–17.

Malone, B. et al. 1996. "A Grim Prognosis for Healthcare." *American Journal of Nursing Survey Results*, November, 40.

Manion, J. 1996. "Understanding the Seven Stages of Change." *RN Magazine*, April, 21.

Manthey, M. 1994. "Issues in Patient Care Delivery." *Journal of Nursing Administration* 24(12): 14–16.

Manuel, P., and Sorensen, L. 1995. "Changing Trends in Healthcare: Implications for Baccalaureate Education, Practice and Employment." *Journal of Nursing Education* 34(6): 248–253.

Margulies, N., and Raia, A.R., eds. 1972. *Organizational Development: Values, Process, and Technology*. New York: McGraw-Hill.

Marks, M. 1994. *From Turmoil to Triumph*. New York: Lexington Press.

Martel, L. 1986. *Mastering Change: The Key to Business Success*. New York: Simon and Schuster.

Martin, R. 1993. "Changing the Mind of the Corporation." *Harvard Business Review*, November/December, 81–94.

Mauer, R. 1996. *Beyond the Wall of Resistance*. Austin, Texas: Bard Books, Inc.

McCloskey, J., and Grace, H. 1997. *Current Issues in Nursing*. 5th ed. New York: Mosby.

McManis, G.L. 1993. "Reinventing the System." *Hospitals and Health Networks*, 5 October, 42–48.

Merisalo, L., ed. 1998. "RN Staff Cuts Due to Managed Care Pressures May Be Costly." *Managed Care Payment Advisor*, March, 1–2.

Miller, J. 1995. "Leading Nursing into the Future." *Harvard Nursing Research Institute Newsletter* 4(3): 5–7.

Morrell, J. 1995. "Turn Your Focus Outside In." *Hospitals and Health Networks*, 5 December, 66.

Organization of Nurse Leaders. 1995. Focus Group Notes. *Nursing Issues*. 29 September.

O'Rourke, M.W. 1996. "Who Holds the Keys to the Future of Healthcare?" *NurseWeek*, 8 January, 1.

Perryman, A. 1998. "Sixteen Ways to Succeed in a New Work Place." *Executive Female*, April, 14.

Pew Health Professions Commission. 1995. "Healthy America: Practitioners for 2005." *Pew Health Professions Report*. Washington, D.C.: Pew Health Professions Commission.

———. 1998. *Pew Health Professions Report*. Washington, D.C.: Pew Health Professions Commission.

Pinto, C. et al. 1998. "Future Trends." *Modern Healthcare*, 5 January, 27–40.

Porter-O'Grady, T. 1994a. "Working with Consultants on a Redesign." *American Journal of Nursing*, October, 33–39.

———. ed. 1994b. *Implementing Shared Governance*. Chapter 7. New York: Mosby.

Prokesch, S. 1993. "Mastering Chaos at the High-Tech Frontier." *Harvard Business Review*, November/December, 135–144.

Public Policy Institute of California. 1996. *Nursing Staff Trends in California Hospitals: 1977–1995*. Sacramento, California: Public Policy Institute of California.

Rich, P.L. 1995. "Working with Nursing Assistants: Becoming a Team." *Nursing 95*, May, 100–103.

Sheehy, B. et al., 1995. "Don't Blink or You'll Miss It." *The Atlanta Consulting Group*, Atlanta, 69–87.

Shelton, K., ed. 1995. *Executive Excellence Magazine*, February.

Sherer, J. 1994a. "Corporate Cultures." *Hospitals and Health Networks*, 5 May, 20–27.

————. 1994b. "Union Uprising: California Nurses React Aggressively to Work Redesign." *Hospitals and Health Networks*, 20 December, 36–38.

————. 1995. "Tapping into Teams." *Hospitals and Health Networks*, 5 July, 32–35.

Shindul-Rothschild, J. et al. 1997. "Ten Keys to Quality Care." *American Journal of Nursing* 97(11): 35–43.

Shubert, D. 1996. "Hospitals Decrease Nurses' Role: Reassign Tasks to Aides." *Los Angeles Times*, 14 July.

Simmons, H. 1998. "The Forces That Impact Healthcare-Quality and Costs." *Healthcare Forum Journal*, January/February, 27–46.

Sokolosky, V. 1996. "Mastering Career Change." *Spirit* (Southwest Airlines), August, 132–33.

Stewart, T. 1993. "Reengineering: The Hot New Management Tool." *Fortune*, 23 August, 41–45.

St. Vincent Hospital. 1994. "CARE 2000: An Approach to Patient Focused Care." Presentation handouts, February 1994.

Teisberg, E. et al. 1994. "Making Competition in Health Care Work." *Harvard Business Review*, July/August, 131–141.

Truscott, J.P., and Churchill, G.M. 1995. "Patient Focused Care." *Nursing Policy Forum* 1(4): 5–12.

Turner, S.O. 1995a. "Stand Out or Lose Out." *Nursing 95*, January, 13–18.

————. 1995b. "Laid Off: Now What?" *Nursing 95*, May, 94–95.

————. 1995c. "Reality Check: It's Time for Nursing to Face the Future." *Hospitals and Health Networks*, 20 August, 20–22.

————. 1996. "Capitation: Are You Ready for It?" *Surgical Services Management*, February, 43–45.

Ulschak, F., and SnowAntle, S.M. 1995. *Team Architecture*. Ann Arbor, Michigan: American College of Healthcare Executives Foundation, Health Administration Press.

Ummel, S. 1997. "Integration." *Healthcare Forum Journal*, March/April, 13–27.

Van, S. 1994. "A New Attitude." *RN Times*, November, 12–13.

Vitale, S. 1995. "Reinventing Your Career." *Executive Female*, September/October, 43–56.

Woodward, H. 1994. *Navigating Through Change*. Berkeley, California: Richard D. Irwin, Inc.

# CHAPTER 9

# Managing Transition

According to Mitchell Marks, people will change either by design or by default (1994). This means you either create a transition plan and strategies or staff will make up their own. It is not uncommon for staff to resort to doing what they have always done, especially under stress. This spells disaster for patient-focused work transformation.

Transition is the "unfreezing" phase of the change process described by Lewin (Marks, 1994). Staff are doing new behaviors they are uncomfortable with and may have limited knowledge of. To have long-term change be successful, employees must enter transition, achieve recovery after transition, and then be able to become revitalized for the next transition phase (Marks, 1994).

This means that for staff, the transition process will only potentially alter existing mental models, and staff will settle into attitudes and behaviors inadvertently reinforced during the transition (Marks, 1994). The actual transition to patient-focused work processes will not necessarily alter mental models. Old attitudes and behaviors may be retained, and therefore new patterns must be created to replace the old ones.

If a transition plan is created and successful transition strategies are implemented, then successful transition will occur. Successful transition will alter mental models of staff behavior. Staff will settle in and rely on attitudes and behaviors reinforced by the design of management. The most effective method to create positive change is to reinforce and design new attitudes and behaviors.

Marks believes that organizations must change the organizational culture of an institution to make transition successful (1994). In reality, patient-focused work transformation is the creation of a new organizational culture. New processes and systems are developed. New ways of organizational structure and function are identified for staff. Employees expect that senior management will assist them in making any transition required in a work setting.

Hospitals have not been particularly good at recognizing this employee expectation. There is essentially a psychological contract between employees and employers, and each has certain expectations of the other. This unwritten contract implies employers' commitment to employees to assist them through transition.

According to Marks, the organization has several opportunities during transition. Transition creates a new organizational "order" (1994). This new organizational focus allows hospitals to resuscitate the human spirit of their employees, who are often left bereft during periods of downsizing. In addition, patient-focused work transformation allows a transition process that enhances work methods and focuses on tasks. This causes a renewal of human resources, so employees can participate in living the vision.

Organizations must recognize employees' need for transition assistance and provide it—especially to middle managers, who must often cope with overwrought employees and are frequently viewed by some staff members as traitors cooperating with changes insisted upon by upper management. Facilities must promote organizational learning and continually support the transition process.

According to Marks, to be successful and prosper, your employees need to be valued and to feel that they are (1994). They also need transition training and positive feedback from both peers and managers, to feel supported and empowered. This means that the organization must focus on collaboration. It must also provide guidance for implementing the patient-focused work transformation vision and strategic plan, by communicating through actions as well as words to every employee. It is helpful to give employees as much information as possible about the organization, including its financial status and specific payer contract expectations as well as strategies for the transition.

Organizations will face challenges to the new organizational order and focus they have created. There will be resistance to change as well as regression to immature or childish behaviors. This will be seen in both managers and staff-level nurses. Employees at all levels in the organization may display powerlessness and victimization, demotivation, and need for crisis management.

Organizations have to be careful to not have limited or constricted communication and to not make use of outmoded systems. Facilities undergoing patient-focused work transformation must be careful not to demonstrate a lack of consensus, especially at the senior management level. Hospitals must commit resources and be committed to endorsing and creating a long-term philosophical change, not just a programmatic "flavor of the month" change. Successfully managing organizational transition during patient-focused work transformation means demonstrating management consensus, committing sufficient resources, allowing innovation, defining clear outcomes and goals, and creating strategies.

Some facilities will design models that encourage and actually demand high levels of staff autonomy in the new roles. Underlying assumptions about this include the belief that all people in the new roles are motivated by freedom to make many of their own work-related decisions, design their own work flow on a daily basis, and be self-directed. These assumptions can be treacherous and tragic during the transition process.

The reality is that during transition, there will only be a few self-directed and empowered staff members. Most managers have a mix of people who are highly motivated and people who are just there to complete their shift and go home. The second category of workers will be resistant to staying for team meetings after work or participating in problem-solving meetings and attending educational sessions even while on duty. Managers and administrators must be understanding of this mindset and assist all types of employees in achieving organizational recovery from transition.

Organizational recovery is the process described by Marks that institutions go through after the initial transition phase (1994). Staying in transition indefinitely is equivalent to maintaining a "crisis management" mode, which no organization can sustain over a long period of time.

Organizational recovery must be linked with the institution's total quality improvement process. Employees must identify what customers want and how to provide it. This will allow for ongoing success of the organization and high patient satisfaction, and is one reason the data collection during patient-focused work transformation is so crucial. It may be most convenient to use written questionnaires to gather feedback from patients, but personal contact after discharge by staff members can allow patients the opportunity to express emotions and offer solutions. Whatever data collection method is used, the results must be shared with the staff.

It is helpful for the facility to draft a recovery plan that is adaptable to the changing environment. This plan will identify the work attributes essential to maintaining performance standards (flexibility, team play, delegation skills), identify workload and cost of any downsized employees, and attempt to minimize group tension and conflict through communication and education following transition.

Organizations must create a context for recovery. Rebuilding trust in uncertain times is difficult; therefore, it is optimal to develop communication strategies during the transition phase that allow the trust between employers and employees to be maintained. The facility must organize work around new organizational order. The new patient-focused system and process designs should be evident in hospital policies, procedures, and daily operations. This also creates an atmosphere of accepting responsibility. All executives, employees, and managers are responsible for failures and successes.

Facilities must be upfront and honest in communicating the new systems to employees. They will maintain employee integrity by focusing on the changing processes and not on employee productivity or cost. Employee tasks, roles, responsibilities, and relationships should be aligned with critical business needs of the organization. It is important for managers to emphasize local design at the unit staff level, not in organization-wide programs. This will succeed because unit employees understand work tasks. This understanding will lead to recovery buy-in on specific units.

Recovery must be led from the top of the organization. The most important resource during organizational recovery is coaching. The most important tools to do so are education and communication. Managers and employees must be motivated from the inside, persuaded in heart and mind, not just convinced by management to change behaviors. It is important for managers to be empathetic and patient. They must allow and encourage venting and grieving, but present other perspectives to offer opportunities for growth. All should anticipate mistakes and allow for "hang time" in between old and new organizational cultures during which acceptance of the new culture will increase. Managers must make a reasonable timeline and set deadlines with input from staff. Management's role is to ensure the organizational change is complete as well as successful.

In order to assist employees through recovery, senior management must understand what employees need in order to recover from transition. According to Marks, employees must understand the benefits of change and see that their work is in alignment with the new organizational order and structure (1994). Employees will need to learn new skills and gain new experience. They need to receive fair rewards, in terms of salary, communication, and support, to participate successfully in the transition and to move through recovery. Employees need to hear the truth and be able to maintain trust and confidence in leadership. To maintain trust, managers must provide open communication. Employees must see managers respond with empathy and consistency to staff going through transition. Managers must treat all employees with fairness and integrity and be able to "walk the walk" and "talk the talk" of transition. Employees must see the organization revitalized from the top down—from the vision and mission through the policies, procedures, and performance expectations of each unit.

## DISCUSSION QUESTIONS

1. Has reengineering been managed well by health care providers in your geographic location? Why or why not?
2. Has reengineering been managed well by nurses in your geographic location? Why or why not?
3. List and explain four strategies for managing reengineering that would likely be successful for nurses in your geographic area.
4. Do you think health care providers should assist nurses in dealing with changes in the workplace? Why or why not?
5. Give examples of behaviors nurses may exhibit if they are not able to cope with changes in the workplace.

**BIBLIOGRAPHY**

Adizes, S. 1993. *Mastering Change*. Pacific Palisades, California: Adizes Institute Publications.

Aiken, L. et al. 1994. "Lower Medicare Mortality among a Set of Hospitals Known for Good Nursing Care." *Medical Care* 32(8), June, 771–785.

American Nurses' Association. 1993. *Nursing's Agenda for Health Care Reform*. Washington, D.C.: ANA Publishing.

———. 1994. *Every Patient Deserves a Nurse*. Brochure. Washington, D.C.: ANA Publishing.

———. 1996. *Registered Professional Nurses and Unlicensed Assistive Personnel*. 2nd ed. Washington, D.C.: ANA Publishing.

American Organization of Nurse Executives. 1996. *Talking Points on Hospital Redesign*. Washington, D.C.: American Organization of Nurse Executives.

Ashton, J., and Fike, R., eds. 1996. *Reengineering for Patient-Focused Care*. Boston: Prescott Publishing.

Austin, N. 1995. "The Skill Every Manager Must Master." *Working Woman*, May, 29–30.

Beyers, M. 1996. "The Value of Nursing." *Hospitals and Health Networks*, 5 February, 52.

Bridges, W. 1980. *Transitions*. Boston: Addison Wesley Publishing.

———. 1988. *Surviving Corporate Transition*. New York: Doubleday.

Butts, J., and Brock, A. 1996. "Optimizing Nursing through Reorganization: Mandates for the New Millennium." *Nursing Connections* 9(4): 5–10.

California Strategic Planning Committee for Nursing. 1996. *Final Report*. Irvine, California: California Strategic Planning Committee for Nursing.

California Nurses Association. Web Site Home Page. http://www.califnurses.org/

Christensen, P., and Bender, L. 1994. "Models of Nursing Care in a Changing Environment." *Orthopaedic Nursing* 13(2): 64–70.

Dracup, K., and Bryan-Brown, C., eds. 1998. "Thinking Outside the Box and Other Resolutions." *American Journal of Critical-Care*, January, 1.

Duck, J.D. 1993. "Managing Change: The Art of Balancing." *Harvard Business Review*, November/December, 109–118.

Flower, J. 1997. "Job Shift." *Healthcare Forum Journal*, January/February, 15–24.

Fralicx, R., and Bolster, C.J. 1997. "Preventing Culture Shock." *Modern Healthcare*, 11 August, 50.

Gray, B.B. 1994a. "Twenty-First Century Hospital Embodies New Concept." *NurseWeek*, 1 April, 1.

———. 1994b. "Changing Skill Mix Reorders Healthcare Delivery System." *NurseWeek*, 2 December, 14.

———. 1995. "Issues at the Crossroads." Parts 1 and 2. *NurseWeek*, 1 October, 1.

Hagland, M. 1995. "Incent Me." *Hospitals and Health Networks*, 5 September, 7.

Hall, G. et al. 1993. "How to Make Reengineering Really Work." *Harvard Business Review*, November/December, 119–131.

Hammer, M., and Champy, J. 1995. *Reengineering the Corporation*. New York: Harper Business.

Hammers, M.A. 1994. "Crystal Ball Gazing with Leland Kaiser." *RN Times*, 5 September, 8–10.

Harrington, C., and Estes, C., eds. 1997. *Health Policy and Nursing*. 2nd ed. Boston: Jones and Barlett.

Izzo, J. 1998. "The Changing Values of Workers." *Healthcare Forum Journal*, May/June, 62–65.

Jaffe, D., and Scott, C. 1997. "The Human Side of Reengineering." *Healthcare Forum Journal*, September/October, 14–21.

Kanter, R.M. 1983. *The Change Masters*. New York: Simon and Schuster.

———. 1990. *When Giants Learn to Dance*. New York: Simon and Schuster.

Katzenbaach, J.R., and Smith, D.K. 1993. *The Wisdom of Teams*. New York: Harper Collins.

Keepnews, D., and Marullo, G. 1996. "Policy Imperatives for Nursing in an Era of Healthcare Restructuring." *Nursing Administration Quarterly* 20(3): 19–31 (spring).

Kemp, V.H. 1995. "Overview of Change and Leadership." *Contemporary Leadership Behavior*. 2nd ed. Boston: Little Brown and Company, 275–282.

Kunen, J. 1996. "The New Hands-Off Nursing." *Time*, 30 September, 55–57.

Lanara, V.A. 1993. "The Nurse of the Future, Role and Function." *Journal of Nursing Management* 1: 83–87.

Larson, C.E., and LaFasto, F.M. 1989. *Teamwork: What Must Go Right, What Can Go Wrong*. Newbury Park, California: Sage Publications.

MacStravic, S. 1997. "Managing Demand: The Wrong Paradigm." *Managed Care Quarterly* 5(4): 8–17.

Malone, B. et al. 1996. "A Grim Prognosis for Healthcare." *American Journal of Nursing Survey Results*, November, 40.

Margulies, N., and Raia, A.R., eds. 1972. *Organizational Development: Values, Process, and Technology*. New York: McGraw-Hill.

Marks, M. 1994. *From Turmoil to Triumph*. New York: Lexington Press.

Martel, L. 1986. *Mastering Change: The Key to Business Success*. New York: Simon and Schuster.

Martin, R. 1993. "Changing the Mind of the Corporation." *Harvard Business Review*, November/December, 81–94.

Mauer, R. 1996. *Beyond the Wall of Resistance*. Austin, Texas: Bard Books, Inc.

McManis, G.L. 1993. "Reinventing the System." *Hospitals and Health Networks*, 5 October, 42–48.

McNeese-Smith, D. 1995. "Leadership Behavior and Employee Effectiveness." *Nursing Management* 24(5): 38–39.

Meissner, J. 1986. "Nurses: Are We Eating Our Young?" *Nursing 86*, March, 52–53.

Morrell, J. 1995. "Turn Your Focus Outside In." *Hospitals and Health Networks*, 5 December, 66.

O'Rourke, M.W. 1996. "Who Holds the Keys to the Future of Healthcare?" *NurseWeek*, 8 January, 1.

Pallarito, K. 1996. "Deloitte Survey Identifies Service Consolidation as Key to Efficiency." *Modern Healthcare*, 24 June, 3.

Pew Health Professions Commission. 1995. "Healthy America: Practitioners for 2005." *Pew Health Professions Report*. Washington, D.C.: Pew Health Professions Commission.

―――. 1998. *Pew Health Professions Report*. Washington, D.C.: Pew Health Professions Commission.

Pinto, C. et al. 1998. "Future Trends." *Modern Healthcare*, 5 January, 27–40.

Porter-O'Grady, T. 1994. "Working with Consultants on a Redesign." *American Journal of Nursing*, October, 33–39.

Prokesch, S. 1993. "Mastering Chaos at the High-Tech Frontier." *Harvard Business Review*, November/December, 135–144.

Public Policy Institute of California. 1996. *Nursing Staff Trends in California Hospitals: 1977–1995*. Sacramento, California: Public Policy Institute of California.

Shelton, K., ed. 1995. *Executive Excellence Magazine*, February.

Sherer, J. 1994. "Corporate Cultures." *Hospitals and Health Networks*, 5 May, 20–27.

Shindul-Rothschild, J. et al. 1997. "Ten Keys to Quality Care." *American Journal of Nursing* 97(11): 35–43.

Shubert, D. 1996. "Hospitals Decrease Nurses' Role: Reassign Tasks to Aides." *Los Angeles Times*, 14 July.

Simmons, H. 1998. "The Forces That Impact Healthcare-Quality and Costs." *Healthcare Forum Journal*, January/February, 27–46.

Stewart, T. 1993. "Reengineering: The Hot New Management Tool." *Fortune*, 23 August, 41–45.

Turner, S. O. 1995a. "Stand Out or Lose Out." *Nursing 95*, January, 13-18.

―――. 1995b. "Laid Off: Now What?" *Nursing 95*, May, 94–95.

―――. 1995c. " Managing Your Transition: Strategies for the Future." *Surgical Services Management*, May, 40–42.

―――. 1995d. "Nurses: Are They the Key to Successful Capitation?" *Capitation and Medical Practice*, December, 1–2.

―――. 1996. "Capitation: Are You Ready for It?" *Surgical Services Management*, February, 43–45.

# CHAPTER 10

# The Nursing Studies: What Are the Implications for Nurses?

> "The implications of changes in the health care environment for the nursing work force are profound in terms of numbers, adequate distribution of skills, and educational preparation. . . . Nursing personnel are an integral component of the health care delivery system, therefore, they are affected directly by these changes" (Davis, 1996, p. 14). These are findings from the most recent national study on the nursing profession in the United States.

Two reports have been generated in the last few years that dramatically affect the future practice of nursing in this country. The National **Institute of Medicine (IOM)** study and the 1998 Pew Health Professions Commission Report both describe future nursing activities and work force needs. Nurses must be aware of what is being reported about their profession to plan their careers accordingly.

## NATIONAL INSTITUTE OF MEDICINE STUDY

It is not surprising that concerns about the fate of nurses are increasing in this new managed health care arena, or that they are reported in the media. Many consumers are aware that within the nursing profession and nursing organizations there is uncertainty and concern about what is happening to nurses, in terms of physical, psychological, and economic well-being. Individual health care givers, professional nursing associations, and labor unions have all expressed concerns that these changes are endangering the quality of patient care, and causing nurses to suffer increased rates of injury, illness, and stress.

Because of these publicized concerns, Congress directed the Secretary of the Department of Health and Human Services (DHHS) to ask the Institute of Medicine (IOM) to undertake a study to determine whether and to what extent there is need for an increase in the number of nurses in hospitals and nursing homes in order to promote the quality of patient care and reduce the incidence among nurses of work-related injuries and stress. For the purposes of that study, Congress defined "nurses" to include registered nurses, licensed practical (vocational) nurses, and nursing assistants (Davis, 1996).

To initiate this legislative mandate, in March 1994, the Division of Nursing of the Health Resources and Services Administration requested that the IOM appoint a committee of experts to undertake an independent objective study as stipulated by Congress (Davis, 1996). In response to this request, the committee explored:

- current levels of quality of care in hospitals and nursing homes;
- the relationship of quality of care or quality of nursing care and patient outcomes to nurse staffing levels and mix of different types of nursing personnel;
- the current supply and demand for nurses, including both American- and foreign-trained nurses, and the current and expected levels of work force participation in that professional group;
- existing ratios of nursing personnel to other measures of demand for health care, such as numbers of patients in hospitals or residents in nursing homes, or numbers of beds, and how those ratios might vary by type of facility, geographic location, or other factors;
- the incidence and prevalence of work-related stress and injuries among nurses in these settings; whether the epidemiology of these problems had been changing in recent years; and whether they differ by type of nursing personnel;
- types and levels of education and training of different types of nurses; and
- the current and projected patient population of the nation, taking into account the aging of the US population, the changing racial and ethnic composition of that population, and the implications of these demo-

graphic shifts for the types of health care providers—especially nurses of various kinds— that will be needed in future years (Davis, 1996).

To address these charges in an organized way, the committee conducted many activities. These activities included:

- reviewing the relevant literature
- analyzing data from various sources
- talking with various experts
- holding public hearings
- obtaining and reviewing written testimony
- conducting site visits
- meeting with professional groups
- commissioning several background papers from experts

In conducting these activities, the committee determined that, although interest and concern among nursing groups about staffing conditions in hospitals and nursing homes is intense, the future needs for nursing services in the overall health care system of the United States are equally critical for planning and policy formulation.

The major findings and conclusions of the committee are outlined and discussed in this chapter. For a complete review of the recommendations and text, please see the IOM Report (Davis, 1996). These findings are extremely important to the profession of nursing and to how we direct our future course of actions. Nursing will not be as successful at carving out a key position at the health care table without considering these issues.

To determine the adequacy of nursing personnel in hospitals and nursing homes, the IOM committee first evaluated the overall supply of nursing personnel in the context of the shifting demand for nursing services. They found that the demand for nurses is increasing and that, although focus is shifting away from hospital care, the largest number of nursing personnel are still working in hospital inpatient settings. The committee also recognized that with the emerging complexity of case mix in nursing homes, the need for professional nursing is much greater now than in the previous years, and will be even greater in the future.

The continuing trends of reducing inpatient hospitalization rates, increased patient acuity in hospitals, and the shift of nursing employment to ambulatory and community-based care settings will have significant implications for registered nurses in hospitals in terms of employment, education, and training. In the future, registered nurses will likely be called upon to fill roles that require increased professional judgment and management of complex systems, with expanded roles and greater clinical autonomy that challenge the traditional boundaries of care settings and role function.

In addition, the nursing home setting is no longer focused only on the chronic and custodial care of long-term residents. In fact, nursing homes are entering into a completely different line of business—providing subacute and transitional care services for patients who would have been kept in hospitals in the past but, with the change toward reduced lengths of stay, are now discharged from hospitals to nursing homes.

These factors raised important questions about the adequacy of RN educational preparation in relation to future RN supply and needs of health care consumers. The IOM committee concluded the aggregate numbers are adequate to meet national needs for the near future, but the RN education mix is not adequate to meet either current or future demands of a rapidly changing health care system.

The committee also acknowledged that nursing services are central to the provision of hospital care. As most nurses have known for years, the reason patients are hospitalized is for the nursing care they require. Every other care-related procedure can be done in an alternative setting by providers outside hospital walls. Nursing care in hospitals takes on additional import now because the increased acuity of patients requires intensive nursing care that involves complex and critical nursing skills. At the same time, the rapidly changing health care environment continues to put pressure on hospitals to contain costs, and the continually rising patient acuity and comorbidity requires innovative and unique ways of redesigning care delivery while maintaining care quality.

Redesign of services is a central strategy used by most hospitals. Most hospitals are driven to redesign by the need to reduce operating costs. There are significant issues involving redesign and restructuring, discussed elsewhere in this book. Many of these issues were analyzed and addressed by the IOM study. The IOM committee also recognized that staff reduction and downsizing is another method used by hospitals to reduce cost, and that organizational changes that facilitate the possibility of better patient outcomes with fewer but more specialized staff may benefit both hospital bottom lines and patient care quality and satisfaction.

The committee also evaluated the need for all caregivers and patients to think about the continuum of care needed over a lifetime rather than only an episode of hospitalization. Central to these changes is the need to help RNs and other health care workers to learn how to plan for patient care prior to the patient being admitted to the hospital, as well as after discharge from the hospital. Faced with this challenge, as well as the need for increased efficiency, many hospitals across the nation have implemented patient-centered care strategies. The concept of patient care organization is discussed elsewhere in this book.

Based on all of these changes in health care delivery, the IOM committee recognized that the organizational transitions required skills and training that many RNs presently do not have. The committee believes that it will be imperative for management, leadership, care-directing, and supervisory skills to be obtained and fostered through various educational programs. The committee also believes that more advanced and broadly trained RNs will be needed in the future. Clinical nurse specialists, nurse practitioners, nurse midwives, and nurse anesthetists are all going to be needed in greater numbers to provide both inpatient and outpatient care in a variety of settings while performing independent and expanded practice roles.

The IOM committee also evaluated the usage of ancillary nursing personnel in hospitals and nursing homes. Almost all hospitals in the United States use some kind of ancillary nursing personnel to assist RNs by providing certain care delivery tasks. Recently, because of the cost limitations faced by hospitals, that nursing assistance role has been changing and expanding. Many facilities are using ancillary nursing personnel to provide increasingly complex care tasks and direct care activities. This has been an area of much emotion and debate for organized nursing labor unions. The result of this increased use of ancillary personnel is increased levels of management, supervision, and oversight of their task delivery by registered nurses, many of whom have not been trained in those types of skills.

By definition, ancillary nursing personnel—specifically, nursing assistants—have less formal education and training than RNs or LPN/LVNs. Currently no national standards exist for minimum training or certification of the ancillary staff members providing care in and employed by hospitals. Several national organizations are working to develop certification criteria and testing processes. Also, no mechanisms exist at present to evaluate or measure the skills competencies of these caregivers or document that they have demonstrated at least a basic mastery of needed skills. The IOM committee has grave concerns about these deficiencies and the potential for adverse impacts on patient care outcomes and quality.

Cultural diversity of the population is a consideration that the committee believes will become increasingly important in the future. The population is not only aging but becoming more racially and ethnically diverse, requiring caregivers with cultural sensitivity and understanding (Davis, 1996).

The committee also expressed concern about the disruptions and frustrations among nursing staff related to changes in the ways hospitals are conducting business. The intensity of testimony and commentaries made the committee members aware of registered nurses' concerns about the issues of future employment, professional role changes, and potential undesirable and unanticipated effects on quality of care. The committee believes that "the harmful and demoralizing effects of these changes on the nursing staff can be mitigated, if not forestalled altogether, with more recognition on the part of the hospital industry that involvement of nursing personnel from the outset in the redesign efforts is critical" (Davis, 1996). The committee also found that "lack of reliable and valid data on the magnitude and distribution of temporary or permanent unemployment, reassignments of existing nursing staff, and similar changes in the structure of nursing employment opportunities greatly hampers efforts at understanding the problems and planning for the future" (Davis, 1996, p. 9).

In addition to evaluating nursing personnel skills and staffing issues, the committee attempted to evaluate and measure quality of care in hospitals. The committee first looked at quality in terms of the overall care quality received by patients in the hospital and then examined the relationship between structural variables, processes, and outcomes of care. The committee believed that ensuring the quality of patient care is central to the mission of health care services in hospitals.

## PEW HEALTH PROFESSIONS COMMISSION REPORT

The Pew Health Professions Commission released a report in April 1998 detailing its suggestions for the downsizing and restructuring of the nursing profession. The commission recommended closing some nursing schools and reducing the number of registered nurses by 20 percent, with almost all of the reduction coming from the ranks of **associate-degree nurses (ADN)**.

The panel also called for ladder-type credentialing of nurses, to support a system of greater professional differentiation among nurse training levels. According to Ed O'Neil, Executive Director of the Pew Commission, different tasks are done by nurses with different levels of training, and salaries vary commensurately with those training levels (Pew, 1998).

Some organizations, such as the California Nurses' Association, see the report as promoting a system that would eliminate the role of the registered nurse at the bedside (CNA web site, June 1998). Other spokespersons of the profession tend to concur with the Pew Commission's findings that these are appropriate responses to managed care. According to Deloras Jones, Director of Nursing for all of Kaiser Permanente's nurses in California, "The best strategy for the nursing profession is to train increasing numbers of master's level **advanced practice nurses** and nurse practitioners, emphasize a four-year baccalaureate training for registered nurses, and concede some lower-level bedside functions for patients to less skilled UAPs." (telephone conversation, April 1998).

In California, the California Strategic Planning Committee for Nursing (**CSPCN**) has determined that additional **BSN** (baccalaureate prepared) **nurses** are required for today's health care system. According to Geraldine Bednash, Executive Director of the American Association of Colleges of Nursing (**AACN**), "It has been our position that the **nurse clinicians** who come out of associate degree and diploma programs are very different from the nurses who come out of baccalaureate programs" (AACN web site, June 1998).

In reality, our health care system now demands clinicians with better education to deal with the complexity of the system and of patient care. Since 1996, the AACN has supported a bachelor of science degree in nursing as the minimum entry level educational foundation for professional nursing practice. Unlicensed assistive personnel will continue to perform bedside duties that do not demand professional training or cognitive skills, and will require supervision by registered nurses at the baccalaureate level.

Patients now require large amounts of technical equipment such as tubes, drains, parental fluids, pain control devices, and physiologic monitoring. Comprehensive pre- and post-hospital planning, intervention, and disease management are foundations of the managed care delivery system. All of this requires coordination, according to the Pew report, and "[c]ritical thinking and higher levels of professional judgement and autonomy will be essential, requiring that a preponderance of baccalaureate-educated nurses be prepared" (Pew, 1998, p. 4).

Skills of even greater complexity are required in ambulatory care settings. Advanced practice nurses have the ability to provide at least 60 percent of essential primary care services, according to the report. "RNs are becoming increasingly responsible for coordinating care for groups of patients across delivery settings, from ambulatory care to home health to hospital. Care management is another role that RNs may be increasingly called upon to perform. Examples include managing care in such areas as diabetes education, pain management, cardiac rehabilitation, disease management, infusion therapy and communicable diseases" (Pew, 1998, p. 5).

According to O'Neil, managed care could be the force that allows nurses to realize their aspirations to greater responsibility and autonomy, as well as freedom from housekeeping and clerical tasks. "Nurses have always felt like they are in a hierarchical system in which their prerogatives and what they could do and what they could contribute was limited by the medical community" (Pew, 1998, p. 6). O'Neil captures nursing's dilemma well when recognizing that nurses are such a large part of the health care system and are at the center of providing care. Nonetheless, they have both a ceiling and floor problem. Although opportunities exist at the ceiling, nurses spend a lot of time defending the floor.

The Pew report envisions nursing care provided in hospitals to be deployed in teams. These teams will comprise different training levels: LVNs; 2-year, 3-year, and 4-year RNs; and master's-level advanced practice nurses. The utilization of the different levels will depend on the choice of each organization and the context of the practice setting (such as differentiated practice). The majority of hospitals will continue to employ unlicensed assistive personnel as members of nursing teams to support RN staff. The UAP are best utilized to replace the time that nurses have traditionally spent on tasks that UAP could perform with adequate training and supervision.

Some hospitals have cut RN staff too far with the use of UAPs and have seen care quality decrease; they are now trying to bring more nurses back to the bedside. The precipitate use of UAPs as a cost saving seems to be abating. Many hospitals have decided not to use UAPs in critical high-level and complex functions. As they have discovered, it costs more money in the long run to deal with untoward outcomes.

## CONCLUSIONS FROM BOTH STUDIES

While both committees heard significant concerns expressed by RNs about how decreased numbers of RNs in staffing mixes negatively impacts care quality, the committees could find little data or factual evidence to support these anecdotal reports. At the same time, both committees noted that there is a lack of systematic and ongoing monitoring and evaluating of the effects on patient outcomes of organizational redesign and reconfiguration of staffing.

The IOM committee recommended that investigation of hospital quality of care warranted increasing and immediate attention. Hospital research data must consider outcome focuses based on process-of-care problems that occur during hospitalization and episodes of care. In addition, hospitals must also collect data and monitor the effects of RN staffing reconfiguration on patient care quality to determine if a causal relationship exists (Davis, 1996).

While both of the reports drew limited conclusions in some areas and made recommendations in other areas, it is crucial for registered nurses to recognize that the comments contained in the report documents will affect the direction, scope, and practice of all levels of nursing care in the future. Expanded nursing roles, increased accountability and health care decision making are certain outcomes. Differentiated practice and increased nursing education expectations and opportunities are probable outcomes as well. Nurses can and should plan for their futures using the findings of these two reports as a guide.

## DISCUSSION QUESTIONS

1. Who are the health care providers most affected by the IOM and Pew Commission reports in your geographic area? Why?
2. What recommendations in the IOM and Pew Commission reports seem most relevant to health care issues for nurses in your geographic area? Why?
3. Are there additional recommendations that should have been made with regard to nursing care by the IOM and Pew Commission reports for your geographic location? What are they? Why are they relevant?

**BIBLIOGRAPHY**

American Academy of Nursing. Goertzen, I., ed. 1990. "Differentiated Nursing Practice into the Twenty-First Century," *Selected Papers from The American Academy of Nursing*. Washington, D.C.: ANA Publishing.

American Association of Colleges of Nursing. Web Site. http://aacn.org/

California Strategic Planning Committee for Nursing. 1996. *Final Report*. Irvine, California: California Strategic Planning Committee for Nursing.

California Nurses Association. Web Site Home Page. http://www.califnurses.org/

Davis, C., ed. 1996. *Nursing Staff in Hospitals and Nursing Homes: Is It Adequate?* National Institute of Medicine. Baltimore: National Academy Press.

Dillon, P. 1997. "The Future of Associate Degree Nursing." *Nursing and Healthcare: Perspectives on Community* 18:1.

Donaho, B., ed. 1996. *Celebrating the Journey: A Final Report on Strengthening Hospital Nursing*. Philadelphia: National Academy Press.

Fosbinder, D. et al. 1997. "The National Healing Web Partnership." *Journal of Nursing Administration* 27:4.

Lanara, V.A. 1993. "The Nurse of the Future, Role and Function." *Journal of Nursing Management* 1: 83–87.

Malone, B. et al. 1996. "A Grim Prognosis for Healthcare." *American Journal of Nursing Survey Results*, November, 40.

Pew Health Professions Commission. 1995. "Healthy America: Practitioners for 2005." *Pew Health Professions Report*. Washington, D.C.: Pew Health Professions Commission.

Pew Health Professions Commission. 1998. *Pew Health Professions Report*. Washington, D.C.: Pew Health Professions Commission.

RN Special Advisory Committee. 1990. *Meeting the Immediate and Future Needs for Nursing in California*. Sacramento, California: State of California.

Shindul-Rothschild, J. et al. 1997. "Ten Keys to Quality Care." *American Journal of Nursing* 97(11): 35–43.

# CHAPTER 11

# Differentiated Professional Nursing Practice: What Is It?

Health care systems are currently undergoing massive changes that will require a nursing work force targeted in its capabilities, efficient in its work, and productive in a cost-effective manner. This necessitates a better match of clinicians with client needs. The evolving health care delivery system demands nursing personnel with specialized skills, competencies and education" (**AONE**, 1996, p. 8).

Chronic and critical fluctuations in the supply of and demand for registered nurses (RNs) represents a direct threat to health care for the people of the United States. In response to that deficit, some states have created nursing advisory committees to develop recommendations for each individual state, the states' Boards of Registered Nursing (BRN), and other appropriate entities to increase the supply and utilization of RNs, as well as to identify projects that demonstrate innovative approaches to providing education and promoting practice.

These advisory committees have addressed a broad range of issues related to education access, program capacity, and public policy implications to ensure adequate nursing services for Americans (AONE, 1996). In response to the final report in California, the California Strategic Planning Committee for Nursing (CSPCN) was formed in 1991 as an unincorporated consortium to begin work on differentiated practice in that state. Other states, including Colorado, Utah, New Mexico, South Dakota, and

Mississippi, have implemented programs designed to address professional differentiated nursing practice.

One of the dilemmas for these groups is that no reliable data resources were available to make an assessment of work force supply and future demand, so CSPCN developed and maintains a dynamic forecasting model to predict the nursing work force that California's people will need for their health care. This model is also in use in several other states. In addition, these states are developing strategic plans to ensure that the supply of nurses meets the demand, and are beginning to develop resources to implement the strategic planning process (CSPCN, 1996).

The development of work force projections in nursing was a difficult and challenging goal. The variety of nursing education programs available throughout the country and the nursing clinicians produced in these programs has resulted in a mix of providers with different sets of skills yet similar role expectations. In addition, the nursing work force supply and demand frequently have been "out of sync" as the health care employment market fluctuated, often with nursing clinician production in the various programs having no relationship to current need (AONE, 1996).

As nursing educators and service representatives debated these discrepancies, it became apparent that the lack of differentiation of nursing roles was a major component of the problem. It was discovered through this process that without differentiated practice, differentiated curricula served no purpose.

Differentiated nursing practice has been a goal of nursing professionals throughout the United States for a long time. "Differentiated practice can be defined as the practice of structuring nursing roles on the basis of education, experience and competence" (AONE, 1996). In 1984, the Kellogg Foundation funded a three-year project entitled the National Commission on Nursing Implementation Project (**NCNIP**). One of the purposes of that project was to facilitate differentiated practice in nursing in response to recommendations by the 1983 Institute of Medicine (IOM) Report, *Nursing and Nursing Education: Public Policies and Private Actions,* and the National Commission on Nursing's (**NCN**) 1983 publication, *Summary Report and Recommendations.* The NCN report recommended that the Midwest Alliance in Nursing develop differentiated practice competencies, and it did produce seminal work on differentiated competencies.

*Bridging the Gap: Articulation in Nursing Programs* was developed jointly by Associate Degree (ADN) and Bachelor Degree (BSN) educators in California. It outlined common curriculum areas for both ADN and BSN programs, and additional content addressed in BSN programs. This study included work from other extant documents, such as the National League of Nursing Council of Associate Degree Programs' *Educational Outcomes of Associate Degree Nursing Programs* (1990) and American Association of Colleges of Nursing's *Essentials of College and University Education for Professional Nursing* (1986).

Implications for the education and training of RNs were identified in relation to increasing levels of professional judgment required in roles in hospital settings, management of complex systems without traditional service boundaries, and increasing clinical autonomy.

While aggregate numbers of RNs may be adequate, educational mix may be inadequate for current and future health care delivery changes. The expanded use of advanced practice nurses (APNs) in hospitals to provide leadership and cost-effective care, testing and certification of ancillary and unlicensed assistive personnel (UAPs), and involvement of nursing personnel in organizational redesign and staffing reconfiguration planning were among the IOM committee's recommendations (Davis, 1996).

The Pew Health Professions Commission released its third report, *Health America: Practitioners for 2005,* in 1995 (Pew, 1995). In addition to recommendations for the education of all health professionals, the Commission made specific recommendations for each health professional group. In their 1998 report, the Pew Health Professions Commission makes numerous recommendations about future nursing work force needs.

Specific recommendations to the nursing profession are related to nomenclature, differentiation of practice, and education program changes. Recommendations included:

- recognition of the value of multiple entry points into the profession;
- identification of a single title for each nursing preparation level and service;
- differentiation of practice responsibilities among nurses from various educational backgrounds (entry-level hospital and nursing home practice for associate degree graduates, hospital-based management and community-based practice for baccalaureate degree graduates, and hospital specialty or independent primary care provider roles for master's degree graduates) and strengthening of career ladder opportunities;

- expansion of master's level practitioner programs and encouragement of federal support for students in the programs;
- development of new models between education and highly integrated health systems;
- recovery of the clinical management role of nursing (Pew, 1995).

Currently, the dynamic health care environment is dramatically shifting the principles that organize the delivery of health care. As managed care organizations have achieved growing prominence as the largest deliverers of health care services, cost-efficiency has become an important principle of health care organizations. Increased focus on utilization of work force resources is causing increased interest in examining the unique skills and knowledge of all health professionals, especially nurses.

The growth in managed care organizations has also generated intense discussion with regard to the size and resource utilization of the acute care sector, the major site of employment for nurses. In 1992, according to the Department of Health and Human Services, almost two-thirds of all professional nurses were employed in hospitals. Currently, few data are available to provide a comprehensive view of how the employment picture has shifted or is continuing to shift. Anecdotal reports of downsizing both hospital proportions of care and the work force in these settings have raised growing concerns about the appropriate skill mix in this environment and the work site transitions that will be necessary in this evolving health care system (AONE, 1996).

## REVOLUTION IS NEEDED IN NURSING EDUCATION

In the midst of this changing health care delivery scenario are nursing education systems that are reexamining the educational programs that prepare basic and advanced practice nurses. These major changes in health care delivery have stimulated continuing changes in nursing education.

Any changes in nursing education must explicitly recognize that a variety of nursing competencies are needed in the health care system and that the variety of educational programs that exist must more economically direct their resources to preparing differentiated graduates. The process of transition to a restructured delivery environment and an education system that prepares nurses for differentiated practice must include all relevant parties. A process that includes both the educators and employers of the nursing work force increases the potential for development of a realistic and acceptable approach to rational work force planning and production.

Demonstration projects are being conducted in a variety of locations across the country that experiment with differentiated learning and practice experiences for nurses. Current efforts can be built upon to enhance nursing students' successes.

In 1988, a statewide initiative was introduced in Colorado as a result of growing concerns about recruitment to nursing as a profession. Representatives of the diverse components of the nursing profession developed two sets of recommendations. First, a statewide plan to facilitate articulation of nursing education programs of various lengths and types was completed. The final goal of the articulation plan was to assist nurses to move from one educational credential to another without unnecessary repetition of learning or curricular experience. Second, a differentiated model for nursing practice was developed to facilitate appropriate utilization of nurses with varying educational credentials and degrees of experience. A differentiated pay scale was recommended by this model to allow appropriate compensation of nurses as career advancement or growth occurred.

A complex set of competency statements, job descriptions, and evaluative tools was developed as part of this experiment. Definitions of competency within each role also were developed to characterize career growth within each distinct role (e.g., the associate degree nurse, the baccalaureate degree nurse, and the master's degree nurse.)

Included in this model was the clear expectation that movement from one role to another required addition of the appropriate degree, although growth within each role was possible without acquiring formal education. Also implicit in this model was the understanding that expertise can be attained within each role. Although this model was described in 1988, wide-scale implementation has not occurred (AONE, 1996).

## THE SIOUX FALLS PROJECT

In a Healing Web Group project site located in Sioux Falls, South Dakota, the most detailed implementation of practice and education reform has been in place for over eight years. This project is the only effort directed at a differentiated educational design. In this project, nursing students in associate and baccalaureate degree nursing programs are educated in concurrent clinical laboratory experience to differentiated roles. At Augustan College's BSN program and the University of South Dakota's ADN program, a collaborative model of differentiated practice has been integrated into their respective baccalaureate and associate degree nursing education programs. Faculty and students use a differentiated curriculum that provides learning experiences specifically targeted to the competencies associated with the two entry-level program types (Koerner and Karpiuk, 1994).

Implementation of this clinical experience is conducted at Sioux Valley Hospital in Sioux Falls, which has incorporated differentiated roles for nursing staff. Associate degree and baccalaureate nursing students are partnered for every clinical experience for one full year. The partnered students work as a team, attend post-clinical conferences, present patient care conferences, and at the end of each semester conduct a seminar with case presentations. Experience with this unique learning activity has confirmed that little differentiated learning had occurred prior to this joint activity.

During the first semester, both the BSN and ADN students have a comfortable level of knowledge for practice in the associate degree nursing role. There is little differentiation in the care activities undertaken by the BSN and ADN students. By the end of the first semester, however, beginning differentiation of roles has been established for these two learner groups. The growth continues into the second semester. With coaching toward differentiated roles, team learning directed at establishing the complementary roles allows development of entry-level competence for differentiated practice. The comparison of roles and movement into the differentiated practice roles is a gradual process that requires students and faculty to explicitly articulate the expectations for differentiated practice.

Implementation of a differentiated practice clinical learning model in Sioux Falls did not require major curricular change. Instead, the process for teaching the content and the environment in which it is taught are the elements that were changed (Koerner and Karpiuk, 1994).

## THE AONE/AACN/NOADN FRAMEWORK

Nurses are more satisfied when their career aspirations and skills match the role responsibilities assumed in ways that optimize their practice. This model allows not only for differentiation of nursing practice but also for the appropriate recognition and rewards along the continuum within each differentiated nursing role (AONE, 1996).

A triad of nursing organizations determined that, once the assumptions and values that are held jointly by education and practice are identified, a framework can provide a unifying thread for mutually agreed-upon goals and process. The American Organization of Nurse Executives, the American Association of Colleges of Nursing , and the National Organization of Associate Degree Nursing Programs created a model framework for differentiating nursing practice.

This AONE/AACN/NOADN framework states the following:

1. A less value-laden terminology to describe nursing roles must be developed.
2. The essence of nursing does not change with setting or role.
3. Nursing is process and not a constellation of tasks. The unique function of this task force should be to focus on process, not on a series of definable tasks.
4. Empowerment of the individual patient or **client** is critical to nursing practice. The individual client or patient makes choices based on information provided by the nurse.
5. Differentiated practice is aimed at improving the quality of care delivered and at achieving the best possible care for a given cost (AONE, 1996).

Continued discussion with regard to titling for differentiated roles must be a part of the process to differentiate education and practice. Three components are essential to the designation of appropriate titles for the roles. First, the titles must be mutually developed. Second, the titles must connote differences, not hierarchical assessments of value. Third, the titles and roles must reflect differentiated nursing practice across a diversified health care environment, in all settings (AONE, 1996).

If the work of defining professional practice and differentiating nursing roles were just beginning today, it would be a relatively straightforward job to design the differentiated roles and education. The staff nurse role, however, for all its variability from place to place and over time, has continued to be treated as a unitary role. As a consequence, nurses currently in the profession, although educated in differentiated programs, have practice in a single staff nurse role. Now that primary nursing and case management have expanded that role, it no longer makes sense to continue to stretch this single role to cover expanded functions.

Moving an existing nursing work force into differentiated practice roles poses several challenges. Staff nurses may be uncertain about the uncharted territory represented by the new roles. Nurses in practice may fear losing value and status earned from expertise gained through years of experience. The turmoil in the health care delivery system business accentuates these uncertainties and fears.

The new skills that will be required in an evolving health care delivery system, and the social environment for the practice of nursing, create a new domain for the profession. This is yet another change for nursing staff who are already leery of and exhausted by change.

According to AONE, three key fundamental strategies are necessary in the management of this transition for nurses. The first requires the maximum utilization of the talents existing in each member of the current nursing work force regardless of the educational credential held. The second requires the application of principles of differentiation and mutually valued practice. It is critical to create roles that are different, not roles that can be perceived as greater or better than another. Also, roles must be created that complement each other at the essence yet differ in the skills required. The third and probably most important strategy relates to the resocialization of nurses to actively value and understand, in a new way, the entirety of nursing's work (AONE, 1996).

This transition requires movement of the profession from a prescriptive task focus to a reflective process focus. Nursing roles will change from simply carrying out tasks prescribed by physicians to evaluating the entire care process for a patient across a specific life span. In the emerging health care environment, which is complex, diverse, and spread across the continuum of care delivery sites, nurses interact with the client or family in multiple settings, responding to ever-changing needs. Nurses, therefore, must be able to examine the problem, the context, and the overall needs and expectations of the clients from their unique perspective. This requires nurses to be clinically competent as well as flexible and imaginative in their provision of nursing care. More importantly, this requires matching the unique capabilities of nursing clinicians with patient care requirements (AONE, 1996).

The differentiated roles within nursing are each separate and distinct entities. Yet each of the differentiated roles is held together by the integrated values or essence of nursing. This model of nursing assumes the need for and existence of each role in a comprehensive health care system. The education and preparation of clinicians for each of these roles must also be distinctively separate but collaborative processes.

To ensure nursing as an integral and permanent component of the future health care system, differentiated nursing practice must be implemented in all health care practice settings and differentiated roles must be taught in LVN, ADN, BSN, and MN education settings as well. All integrated nursing roles are necessary to meet the needs of the future health care system— i.e., to provide high-quality, comprehensive, cost-effective care to all patients, in all settings. Initially, differentiation of nursing roles could be based on education, experience, and choice. Differentiated practice pilot sites will be developed and curriculum revisions processed. As the education and practice settings evolve to reflect differentiated practice roles, differentiation will occur through education.

## DIFFERENTIATED PRACTICE FOR THE FUTURE

In the changing health care environment, the hospital will no longer be the center of the health care delivery system. Regional networks of health care facilities will be formed. The patient will move throughout the system from one setting to another and encounters will go beyond one episode of illness and encompass the entire life span. Due to these changes in the health care arena, the model of differentiated practice must be implemented in varied health care delivery sites in which nursing roles can move across environments or from one setting to another.

Current efforts toward differentiated education and practice must be supported. Continued expansion of differentiated practice and education must be reviewed to avoid previous shortcomings of differentiation experiments.

In addition, alternative means must be developed to implement these models in geographic areas in which both ADN and BSN programs do not exist. This would include adoption of long-distance learning modes such as satellite telecommunication, and the use of technologies to provide joint learning experiences.

## DISCUSSION QUESTIONS

1. Has professional differentiated practice been implemented in your geographic area? If so, how has it been implemented?
2. Is differentiated nursing practice an appropriate method of creating nursing functions? Why or why not?

3. Which are the most prevalent degrees offered by schools of nursing in your geographic area? ADN? BSN?

## BIBLIOGRAPHY

Aiken, L. et al. 1994. "Lower Medicare Mortality among a Set of Hospitals Known for Good Nursing Care." *Medical Care* 32(8), June, 771–785.

American Academy of Nursing. Goertzen, I., ed. 1990. "Differentiated Nursing Practice into the Twenty-First Century." *Selected Papers from The American Academy of Nursing.* Washington, D.C.: ANA Publishing.

American Association of Ambulatory Care Nurses. 1996. *Standards for Ambulatory Care Nursing.* Aliso Viejo, California: AACN.

American Association of Colleges of Nursing. 1995. *Essentials of Masters Education for Advanced Practice Nursing.* Unpublished.

American Association of Colleges of Nursing, American Organization of Nurse Executives, and National Organization for Associate Degree Nursing. 1995. *A Model for Differentiated Nursing Practice.* Washington, D.C.: AACN.

———. 1996. *Differentiated Practice Model Framework.* Alisa Viejo, California: AACN Publishing.

American Association of Critical-Care Nurses. 1996. "Decision Grid for Delegation." Staffing Tool Kit. Aliso Viejo, California: AACN Publishing.

American Nurses' Association. 1985. *Code for Nurses.* Washington, D.C.: ANA Publishing.

———. 1993. *Nursing's Agenda for Health Care Reform.* Washington, D.C.: ANA Publishing.

———. 1994. *Every Patient Deserves a Nurse.* Brochure. Washington, D.C.: ANA Publishing.

———. 1995. *Nursing's Social Policy Statement.* Washington, D.C.: ANA Publishing.

———. 1996a. *Registered Professional Nurses and Unlicensed Assistive Personnel.* 2nd ed. Washington, D.C.: ANA Publishing.

———. 1996b. *Scope and Standards of Advanced Practice Registered Nursing.* Washington, D.C.: ANA Publishing.

American Organization of Nurse Executives. 1996. *Talking Points on Hospital Redesign* Washington, D.C.: American Organization of Nurse Executives.

Bayley, E. et al. 1997. "Preparing to Change from Acute to Community Based Care." *Journal of Nursing Administration* 27:5.

Beckham, J. 1996. "The Beginning of the End for HMOs." *Healthcare Forum Journal.* November/December, 44–47.

Bernard, L. and Walsh, M. 1996. *Leadership: The Key to Professionalization of Nursing.* New York: Mosby.

Beyers, M. 1996. "The Value of Nursing." *Hospitals and Health Networks*, 5 February, 52.

Burns, J. 1993. "Caring for the Community." *Modern Healthcare*, 8 November, 30–33.

Butts, J., and Brock, A. 1996. "Optimizing Nursing through Reorganization: Mandates for the New Millennium." *Nursing Connections* 9(4): 49–58.

California Strategic Planning Committee for Nursing. 1996. *Final Report*. Irvine, California: California Strategic Planning Committee for Nursing.

California Nurses Association. Web Site Home Page. http://www.califnurses.org/

Christensen, P., and Bender, L. 1994. "Models of Nursing Care in a Changing Environment." *Orthopaedic Nursing* 13(2): 64–70.

Davis, C., ed. 1996. *Nursing Staff in Hospitals and Nursing Homes: Is It Adequate?* National Institute of Medicine. Washington, D.C.: National Academy Press.

Fosbinder, D. et al. 1997. "The National Healing Web Partnership." *Journal of Nursing Administration* 27:4.

Harrington, C., and Estes, C., eds. 1997. *Health Policy and Nursing*. 2nd ed. Boston: Jones and Barlett.

Koerner, J.G., and Karpiuk, K.L. 1994. *Implementing Differentiated Nursing Practice: Transformation by Design*. Gaithersburg, MD: Aspen Publishers, Inc.

Lanara, V.A. 1993. "The Nurse of the Future, Role and Function." *Journal of Nursing Management* 1: 83–87.

Manthey, M. 1994. "Issues in Patient Care Delivery." *Journal of Nursing Administration* 24(12): 14–16.

Manuel, P., and Sorensen, L. 1995. "Changing Trends in Healthcare: Implications for Baccalaureate Education, Practice and Employment." *Journal of Nursing Education* 34(6): 248–253.

McCloskey, J., and Grace, H. 1997. *Current Issues in Nursing*. 5th ed. New York: Mosby.

McNeese-Smith, D. 1995. "Leadership Behavior and Employee Effectiveness." *Nursing Management* 24(5): 38–39.

Meissner, J. 1986. "Nurses: Are We Eating Our Young?" *Nursing 86*, March, 52–53.

Miller, J. 1995. "Leading Nursing into the Future." *Harvard Nursing Research Institute Newsletter* 4(3): 5–7 (summer).

Miller, M., ed. *Colorado Differentiated Practice Model for Nursing*. Colorado School of Nursing. Unpublished.

National Commission on Nursing Implementation Project. 1986–87 documents.

Neighbors, M., and Monahan, F. 1997. "Are ADNs Prepared to Be Home Health Nurses?" *Nursing and Healthcare: Perspectives on Community* 18:1.

Organization of Nurse Leaders. 1995. Focus Group Notes. *Nursing Issues*. 29 September.

Pew Health Professions Commission. 1995. "Healthy America: Practitioners for 2005." *Pew Health Professions Report*. Washington, D.C.: Pew Health Professions Commission.

———. 1998. *Pew Health Professions Report*. Washington, D.C.: Pew Health Professions Commission.

Public Policy Institute of California. 1996. *Nursing Staff Trends in California Hospitals: 1977–1995.* October. Sacramento, California: Public Policy Institute of California.

RN Scope of Practice. California Business and Professions Code, sec. 2725.

RN Special Advisory Committee. 1990. *Meeting the Immediate and Future Needs for Nursing in California.* Sacramento, California: State of California.

Shindul-Rothschild, J. et al. 1997. "Ten Keys to Quality Care." *American Journal of Nursing* 97(11): 35–43.

Wesorick, B. "Standards: On the Cutting Edge or Over the Cliff?" *Notes on Clinical Practice, 1990s.* Unpublished paper.

# CHAPTER 12

# Managed Care Strategies for the Future

There are specific care management strategies that have been developed and are evolving within the managed care delivery system. Aggressive acute care discharge planning works hand in hand with case management and disease management strategies to provide appropriate health care across the health-illness continuum.

## AGGRESSIVE ACUTE CARE DISCHARGE PLANNING

Discharge planning is a hospital-based function. It is used to assist the hospital in fulfilling its responsibility to employ discharge planners who will help patients arrange for safe and appropriate care after a hospital admission. Discharge planners interview the family and obtain information about the care required by the patient following hospital discharge. The discharge planner will determine what services a patient may require after discharge for continued care, such as home care, and will arrange for those services to be delivered to the patient. The discharge planner will then make all the necessary arrangements for the patient to obtain the care.

If patients require transfer to another type of facility, such as a rehabilitation or long-term care facility, the discharge planner will contact the new facility and set up the actual transfer process. The discharge planner will often inform the patient's family of the transfer order from the physician. Patients cannot be transferred unless they are medically stable and able to be safely transferred. This is federally mandated to avoid inappropriate "dumping" of undesirable patients—those without financial resources or those with social difficulties such as homelessness.

Specific information about discharged patients is required to be given to the receiving facility. Special documentation and patient records are mandated to be completed prior to transfer. Patients and families must be informed of the discharge or request for transfer and agree that it may take place. There are specific instructions mandated by Medicare and other federal and state agencies that must be included in transfer documents and discharge notices of patients.

Discharge planners facilitate all types of services required by patients at any type of facility. They interact with all care providers, including nurses and physicians caring for the patient. Discharge conferences are often scheduled on hospital units so specific discussion can take place. Patient and family needs can be discussed by all caregivers. All health care professionals and therapists as well as the physicians caring for the patient take part in these discussions.

Discharge planners need to be skilled in written and oral communication, conflict management, negotiation, risk-taking, critical thinking, planning, coordinating, and developing creative options. Nurses who enjoy finding innovative solutions to problems may enjoy this type of nursing.

## CASE MANAGEMENT

Case management is a founding principle of managed care. Case management is the axis upon which all other managed care functions rest. Everyone in hospitals, HMOs, and PPOs seems to be focusing on case management. The term is thrown around in most health care settings, but many nurses are unclear as to the meaning and value of this care method. There are several different definitions of case management, and as the field grows, many more are likely to be added.

In 1995, the Case Management Society of America defined case management as a collaborative process that assesses, plans, implements, coordinates, monitors, and evaluates options and services needed to meet a person's health needs. The case manager uses communication and the resources available to promote high-quality, cost-effective outcomes (Zander, 1998). The American Nurses' Association definition includes the goals of enhancing quality of life and decreasing fragmentation of care (1996a).

William J. DeMarco and Jennifer Marx outline principal functions of case management as discussed in a recent article in *Managed Care Pay-*

*ment Advisor* (Merisalo, 1998). The principal functions of case management include:

1. Screening: This identifies those in the targeted population who need case management. It requires asking patients a series of questions to determine the potential risk of high utilization of services.
2. Assessment: This measures patients' physical, mental, social, and clinical status. It is distinguished by a comprehensive, multidimensional, patient-centered approach to evaluating patients' situations and needs. In addition, the assessment should include the adequacy of health services and services from family and friends in meeting patients' needs.
3. Care planning: The assessment is used as a guide to develop a plan for care. This plan indicates the type of proposed services needed and the roles of community agencies and family members.
4. Implementation: Case managers assist clients in gaining needed services according to the care plan. Case managers may either refer clients to the services or, if given fiscal authority, purchase services on behalf of the client.
5. Monitoring: Case managers monitor and report both the progress of the client and the performance of service providers.
6. Reassessment: This occurs at established intervals—every six months, for example. Or it may occur in conjunction with an event that changes a patient's functional status, such as hospitalization (Merisalo, 1998).

According to DeMarco and Marx, the bottom line is that case management allows providers, patients, and patients' families to be actively involved in ongoing care needs. It anticipates potential risks for patients, allowing providers to intervene to minimize those risks for patients.

This type of intervention benefits patients in terms of care and outcomes. Providers benefit by gaining professional satisfaction as well as financial reward by minimizing exposure to risks. In addition, managed Care Organizations (MCOs) that wish to be involved in managed Medicare contracting will have to use case management. Managed Medicare demands a case management approach. In a fee-for-service environment, there is little incentive to adapt the principles of managing health care risks. But that is exactly what must happen in a managed care market.

The good news for nurses is that case management is well-suited for nurses. Take a look at the six principal functions of managed care outlined above. They sound remarkably similar to the nursing process. Nurses are the health care profession most familiar with the functions of case management. They are also likely the most appropriate to act as case managers, as nurses already routinely manage, coordinate, and direct all aspects of patients' hospitalizations. It is an easy addition to bring management of patients outside hospitals and disease management to these nurses' expertise.

According to Karen Zander, RN, MN, CN, FAAN, co-founder of the Center for Case Management in Natick, Massachusetts, the definition of case management is clear, even though there are numerous models and methods that hospitals can use to provide the case management function. The definition of case management, according to Zander, is "a clinical system in which an individual or group is accountable for coordinating patient care across a continuum or episode" (1998).

While that definition remains stable, case management models are evolving as more and more risk is assumed by providers. Zander believes there is an enormous amount of confusion on the part of organizations about which model will best fit them. In an effort to assist facilities in deciding which case management model would work best for them, Zander developed a decision-making tool based on evolving components of the case management roles.

The resulting decision-making framework (Zander, 1998) identifies a four-step case management evolution. Zander defines the four phases, or levels of risk, as shown in Exhibit 12–1.

Zander believes that the farther from the acute care level organizations go with financial risk, the more advanced practice–skilled people are needed, with higher degrees, wider skill sets, and more complex interpersonal skills.

Case management is not a new concept. It has been practiced for almost 100 years. Various public health, insurance, and rehabilitation settings have used case management to reduce medical care costs. Because providers and managed care organizations have recently embraced case management as an effective cost-containment strategy, the field has seen explosive growth. Case management has been used in hospitals since the early 1980s to provide discharge planning for patients, and is now utilized in outpatient, home care, subacute, and community service settings.

Case management can be practiced by several different types of practitioners. The desired background of the case manager depends on the type of agency or program, the population served, and the knowledge level required to perform the role. Case management is currently being practiced

**Exhibit 12–1** Decision-Making Tool

1. Acute Care: At this level, utilization review and discharge planning are no longer separate. Both roles are merged into case management in an attempt to control resources used relevant to doctors' orders and planning for discharge. The concern is with levels of care—i.e., floor care versus ICU. It matches resources to reimbursement.

2. Episode: Medicare drove case management to this level by identifying a discrete episode of care as a new level of financial risk. The financial risk is that there is no reimbursement for extended length of stay; the clinical risk is a lack of coordinated, consistent care, which may compromise outcomes. This is the level at which clinical pathways become useful, and case managers are often assigned to manage them.

3. Continuum/integrated health systems: This level of risk involves more managed care contracting and the need for controlling the environment outside the acute care setting. Although hospitals and other types of providers are merging and/or affiliating into systems, there is usually little continuity between facilities. Also, the complex patients found in this level need management of their transitions between the various levels of care. This level requires clinical management, not paperwork management, and as it involves the investment of more money to be effective, it is not an area of cost savings.

4. Physician practice/community: Capitation is used at this level, and groups of patients must be case managed primarily through physician practices. The financial risk is to manage the per member/per month dollars so that patient care is provided at the lowest level of cost while still providing quality of life and the highest possible level of functioning. Ultimately, population management in the community is the goal, with case management functions being replaced by patient self-management over time.

*Source*: Courtesy of Case Management Center, South Natick, Massachusetts.

by registered nurses, social workers, and therapists. Case management also requires broadening roles and responsibilities of direct care providers in relation to the case management role and function.

The case management process consists of six steps: assessment, planning, implementation, coordination, monitoring, and evaluation. This sounds a lot like the good old nursing process we all learned in nursing school! Nurses already perform most of these steps in patient care, but case management extends the process to include all health care coverage, the family, and the community.

The case manager must be familiar with eligibility criteria for the various services that can be used for patients' physical, mental, emotional, social, vocational, and community integration needs. This role requires that case managers understand the overall treatment plan for each patient, health care delivery systems and networks, reimbursement, legal and ethical issues, and the breadth of community resources available. Case management also requires analysis of costs and benefits of treatment options (Federwisch, 1998; Zander, 1998).

Case management requires skills in critical thinking, communication, negotiation, and collaboration. Critical thinking is a scientifically based process used for gathering, synthesizing, prioritizing, analyzing, and evaluating information. Critical thinking is essential for effective problem solving and decision making. Nurses giving direct care usually possess effective critical thinking skills. Common difficulties in using the critical thinking process are making incorrect assumptions, jumping to conclusions, failing to validate accuracy or reliability of information, acting on incomplete information, and reaching illogical conclusions (Federwisch, 1998).

Communication is the ability to send and receive information in verbal or written form. Case managers must be excellent communicators. They must be able to work effectively with a range of people to carry out the case management plan and achieve the health outcomes desired. Obtaining truthful, accurate information from multiple sources requires strong interpersonal skills with the patient, family, provider(s), and payer. Both critical thinking skills and interpersonal communication skills are used in every step of the case management process.

An additional role of the case manager is patient advocacy. This is a key role, because case managers are the liaison between the health care provider and the payer, and often must speak on behalf of the patient. Case managers also advocate for patients by empowering patients with education about their care and involving them in the recovery and outcomes. Case managers make decisions and recommendations after reviewing all aspects of the care situation. To be most effective, case managers must remain objective and have a high level of credibility and accountability.

In many settings, case managers use multiple components of the case management process simultaneously—it is not a linear, step-by-step process. Different activities occur in more than one area at a time, especially in complex cases. For example, a patient who has undergone cardiac bypass surgery and is recovering well from the surgery may be in the monitoring phase for physical recovery, but in the assessment phase for psychological and vocational issues.

Occasionally, unexpected changes significantly affect treatment and recovery, and case managers need to go back to the assessment phase before proceeding with alternative planning. The processes of monitoring, evaluation, and assessment are used over and over to develop a dynamic case management plan, with strategies that adjust to changing needs.

Assessment is the process of collecting relevant information about a person's current health situation to identify needs and create a plan. Evaluation measures the quality and outcomes of products and services and is done to determine whether the action or plan is producing the desired result (Federwisch, 1998). Assessment and evaluation occur in tandem throughout the case management process.

The type and depth of assessment depend on the patient's medical condition, the circumstances of the case, and the outcome-based goal of case management. Case managers identify all factors likely to significantly influence the patient's recovery or treatment. These types of factors include age; sex; lifestyle choices; medication usage; other medical conditions; psychological, mental, emotional, or social factors; and family influences. Case managers will assess the patient's and family's understanding of the diagnosis and prognosis as well as their expectations. In addition, case managers can identify abnormal coping patterns, unusual family dynamics, or other potential problems during recovery.

Objective observation, physical examination, subjective interviews, and medical records all yield valuable information. Other people familiar with the patient such as family, friends, employers, and caregivers can also be sources of information. In addition to physical assessment findings, the case manager must also research the history and course of the problem, duration of symptoms, effective and non-effective approaches thus far, and the patient's receptivity to various treatments and approaches.

The goal of the case manager is to obtain up-to-date information about the patient. Case managers must review and evaluate medical records and reports for reliability, credibility, and validity. Large amounts of information must be consolidated, organized, and classified to identify patterns, determine pertinence, and decide what additional information, if any, is required. Information from many sources is compared and clarified.

Case managers must also assess and evaluate the financial aspects of patients' care. They gather information about patients' benefits, identifying who is responsible for payment and if the coverage is adequate. They start processes and anticipate barriers. Case managers can make referrals when patients are eligible for other types of services or can assist the patient to self-refer. The case manager can explore alternative sources of care when a patient needs a service for which he or she is not covered. Case managers also assess and evaluate costs and benefits of various care options.

It is essential for case managers to know about any issues that might affect the patient's recovery, such as home support, physical and environmental barriers, occupation, educational level, access to resources and support, previous health care experiences, learning barriers, language barriers, goals, fears, and concerns. Reassessment in all these areas occurs periodically as the issues and circumstances change.

The case manager determines whether the activities conducted have produced the anticipated effect during the evaluation step. If the anticipated effect of the activities has not occurred, the case manager can explore the reasons with the patient. Evaluation can influence decisions about further activities, plans, and resource allocations. Case managers must continually evaluate patients' responses to treatments, approaches, and providers, as well as evaluate how the treatment plan affects the physical, mental, and emotional aspects of recovery. Case managers must also evaluate the cost and appropriateness of the frequency and duration of treatments according to the patient's circumstances and progress, and the actual outcomes achieved compared to the expected outcomes. As case managers realize a patient is not making progress toward anticipated outcomes, they must determine why and take steps to resolve the problem or adjust the goal.

Successful evaluation requires knowing what to look for and asking the right questions, as well as a willingness to correct or redirect actions according to what the evaluation indicates. Information for evaluation includes clinical data, physical data, functional improvement, patient satisfaction, provider input, and progress toward goals. Case managers need to understand the normal and anticipated rate of progress to judge whether the service provided or resource used is of value to a given patient.

Planning is the process of setting up specific objectives, goals, and actions to meet identified needs; implementation is putting that plan into action

(Zander, 1998). The plan should be time-specific, whether the goal is to return the patient to work, discharge to home, or manage a chronic illness.

A case management plan is built on information gleaned from the assessment and evaluation. The plan considers the patient's medical condition, psychological status, social support, and expectations about what is reasonable and realistic given the constraints of a patient's situation. Case management plans include all physical and psychological care aspects as well as coordination of service delivery and resources. In addition, the plan must consider the requirements of patients' insurers and reimbursement criteria. Insurance coverage and benefit information must be investigated and included in the case management plan to ensure that patients are getting the most out of their insurance plan and that there are enough resources to carry out the plan.

The case management plan should contain specific actions, including steps, sequencing, duration, and frequency. Developing a case management plan that is acceptable and agreeable to all involved parties requires complex skills in communication, negotiation, and collaboration. Case managers must check with providers for available services, with payers to ensure that payment is covered and to meet authorization guidelines, and with family members who will take an active role in care provision.

Case managers also facilitate and initiate action as needed, thereby functioning as change agents. The case manager may contact providers to discuss the plan and confirm a certain provider's part in the plan. Case managers may also spend time facilitating care, eliminating barriers to care, and ensuring access to services. They make referrals and link patients to appropriate programs. To make patient compliance more likely, case managers also provide patient education that reinforces instructions from care providers and provides information about resources.

Case managers organize, integrate, modify, and secure the necessary resources to accomplish case management goals and plans. It is the case manager's responsibility to ensure smooth and efficient follow-through of the plan. This accountability includes coordinating as well as monitoring patients' physical and psychological care, medical status and condition, availability of providers to provide agreed-upon services, patients' satisfaction with those services, and the patients' progress toward individual goals of the plan.

Case managers use tools such as clinical pathways or flow sheets to track all the activities and progress. Clinical pathways aid in communication, monitoring, and coordination of care. Case managers determine whether clinical pathway guidelines are appropriate or require modification for specific patients. Some facilities include case managers in clinical pathways' expectations, while other institutions require case managers to oversee the clinical pathways' utilization.

Case managers also make referrals and follow up to ensure that services are progressing as planned. Case managers also communicate pertinent information and changes to the appropriate people, including the patient, physician, other health care professionals, and family members. A case manager is responsible for keeping everyone involved in a patient care plan up-to-date and informed, and for communicating with the payer or claims representative to ensure timely authorization and smooth processing of patient claims.

One of the more important roles for case managers is to communicate with payers: to verify that payer requirements and reimbursement issues are handled and to keep payers updated so that delays or conflicts do not negatively impact patient care or care outcomes. Case managers also coordinate the scheduling of tests and referrals, and gather information from numerous sources at regular intervals. This allows the case manager to verify that the treatment plan is being followed and that everyone is on track. These regular reviews occur daily, weekly, or monthly, and are done with patients, providers, or family members.

Monitoring can reveal barriers to patient compliance such as resource allocation, cultural issues, lack of transportation, or scheduling conflicts. Routine monitoring allows case managers to identify problems early so that adjustments can be made quickly without jeopardizing patient care or patient outcomes.

Case managers are also responsible for making sure that facility discharges are timely, appropriate, and handled efficiently. In some cases, the manager needs to set up services that will provide for patients' needs after they leave a facility or program. Some case managers are responsible for their patients' care and outcomes for only a limited time, such as during a hospitalization. Others follow patients through the entire care continuum from hospitalization to home, outpatient, or subacute care phases.

The evolving health care system demands coordination, efficiency, and effectiveness while containing cost and resource outlays. Nurses who can navigate the complex health care delivery systems can help patients get the care they need. They can advocate for patient education, wellness, and prevention services. They can advocate for resources, access, and smooth transition for patients along the care continuum. Case management offers nurses a way to combine clinical knowledge, communication skills, and nursing process skills in a variety of settings.

## DISEASE MANAGEMENT: THE NEW HEALTH CARE INDUSTRY

Disease management is one of the newest trends in health care. While few groups can really define it, everyone from retail pharmacies to home care companies claims to be involved in it. Few tangible outcomes statistics exist yet, but it is a strategy that is here to stay.

Disease management is not just another industry "flavor-of-the-month" program. Health care is being driven toward a disease management strategy in order to survive economically. Disease management is regarded as a valuable method to improve both clinical and economic outcomes of care (McKinnon, 1996).

Controlling rising health care costs while maintaining care quality has been a major goal for US health care in the past decade. The traditional system, as described in Chapter 3, focuses on providing acute episodic care in a fragmented delivery system involving numerous players. Twenty-five percent of health care dollars go toward administrative costs. Five percent of the sickest patients spend 60 percent of the health care dollars (McKinnon, 1996).

With technological advances, many patients with diseases that once were incurable are now living longer, but at a high cost. Expensive diseases such as AIDS, diabetes, cancer, and renal failure consume a disproportionate share of already limited health care costs.

Larger numbers of aging Americans consume large amounts of health care dollars. Elderly patients use about four times as much medical care as those under age 65, because they are ill more often, recover more slowly, and have simultaneous illnesses.

Health care payers are motivated to manage these expensive patients due to rising health care costs. Case management strategies target high-cost, complex patients while attempting to provide continuity of care and cost management. These types of strategies include management of the costs of individual health care components such as hospitalization, laboratory tests, and drug charges. Unfortunately, reducing costs of one health care component leads to the potential of increasing costs in other areas.

For example, if there is a reduction in the number of drugs available to treat diseases, the drug use declines; however, nursing home and emergency room visits may increase, thereby actually raising overall health care costs. Disease management avoids these cost potholes.

Disease management is a strategy to help manage the quality and cost of care by targeting groups of high-cost patients. Disease management has been defined as a comprehensive, integrated approach to care that focuses on the natural course of disease and emphasizes treatments designed to address an illness with maximum effectiveness and efficiency (McKinnon, 1996). Targets for disease-state management are usually high-cost, chronic diseases that may result in costly complications if not treated properly. Patients are educated to manage their own outpatient drug therapy— a cornerstone of disease management. This promotes both improved disease control and better quality of life for the patient.

Communication between patients, caregivers, and health care professionals is critical to success with disease management. Information is relayed between different parts of the health care delivery system to provide efficient and effective "seamless" care. Patients require extensive education and training so that they can become empowered to manage their own disease state. Cost information must be monitored as well, so that therapeutic and appropriate decisions are also made cost-effectively.

Development of disease care protocols, similar to critical pathways, is one method used to streamline and standardize care. Guidelines defining best practices and clearly outlining roles of all caregivers on the health care team allows care to be delivered more efficiently. Integrated information management systems that allow computerization of the critical pathways along with outcome and cost data are extremely valuable.

Disease management is a long-term strategy and commitment to patients with chronic diseases. These patients may not be cured by disease management, but the benefits include long-term disability reductions, avoidance of drug-related problems, and improved quality of life.

The concept of disease management is a paradigm shift away from treating patients episodically when they are sick to developing long-term strategies to help keep them well. For example, asthmatic patients can be trained to monitor their breathing patterns by measuring "peak flows" and adjust their medication accordingly. Diabetic patients can be trained to monitor blood glucose values and adjust their diet and insulin dosage.

---

### Chronic Diseases for Disease Management Approach

Types of chronic diseases that are successful with a disease management approach, and expensive for traditional health care delivery include:

- angina
- arthritis
- asthma
- cancer
- congestive heart failure
- cystic fibrosis
- depression
- diabetes

- hemophilia
- high blood pressure
- high cholesterol
- HIV/AIDS
- migraine headache
- osteoporosis
- renal failure

---

Congestive heart failure patients can monitor weight; an increase generates a home health visit, medications, and follow-up. These types of interventions put patients in control of their own diseases. Patients who are educated about basic concepts of managing their disease can safely monitor their own symptoms, and institute treatment promptly when needed. Hospitalizations are minimized and so are days missed from work and school. Patients report improved self-esteem and a sense of being in control. Often other health-related behaviors are also improved, such as diet, exercise, and avoidance of tobacco.

Medication compliance is a cornerstone of disease management. Noncompliance causes medication to fail almost 50 percent of the time, at a cost estimate of $100 billion annually (McKinnon, 1996). It is estimated that noncompliance with medication causes 10 percent of hospitalization and 23 percent of nursing home admissions. Potential benefits in cost and outcomes can be achieved if medication compliance can be improved through a disease management program.

Patients must be educated as to the importance of medication compliance. Failing to address their concerns can lead to noncompliance. Health care professionals must teach patients about the purpose of medication therapy, how to use medication properly, and where to get assistance. Medication regimens must be suited to the individual, and patients will often become noncompliant if the regimens are too complex or inconvenient.

Patients can be trained to manage minor adverse effects independently as well as understand severe medication reactions and the need for prompt and immediate medical intervention. Often medications for chronic diseases such as diabetes or hypertension do not make patients feel better. Patients may discontinue medication if they do not understand the importance of the drug to improve the long-term outcome of their disease, or if they perceive the costs as too high. Patients may have unrealistic expectations about new medications, believing these will cure the disease. In fact, many new medications do not cure the disease they control, but rather keep disease symptoms at bay. Telephone follow-up is helpful in promoting compliance and in providing an ongoing open channel for addressing questions and concerns. Written information is also usually given to patients for reinforcement.

Establishing a disease management program requires collaboration of all health care disciplines across the care continuum. Payers and managed care entities are becoming involved in disease management, as are pharmaceutical companies.

Disease management programs are valued by health care providers and payers because they allow costs and outcomes to be identified for high-risk groups of patients. Disease management can be used within the arsenal of strategies to reduce health care costs of managing chronic disease patients. Disease management is not only an important health care opportunity, but a means of improving quality of life and health outcomes for patients.

## DISCUSSION QUESTIONS

1. Are nurses performing case management functions in your geographic area? Why or why not?
2. Are case management functions an extension of the role of the registered nurse, or are they within the role and therefore should be included in all education programs? Why or why not?
3. What applications do you see for case management in your geographic area that are not currently case managed? Why?
4. Does your local health care delivery system have a disease management component? Why or why not?

5. What types of diseases and populations in your local geographic area would benefit from disease management strategies?
6. What are the barriers/benefits to disease management in your local geographic area?
7. Define discharge planning in your geographic location. Is it successful as utilized? Why or why not?
8. Identify and explain the differences among discharge planning, case management, and utilization review nursing functions.
9. Why are discharge planning and utilization review important functions for health care providers?

## BIBLIOGRAPHY

American Association of Colleges of Nursing. 1995. *Essentials of Masters Education for Advanced Practice Nursing*. Unpublished.

American Nurses' Association. 1993. *Nursing's Agenda for Health Care Reform*. Washington, D.C.: ANA Publishing.

————. 1994. *Every Patient Deserves a Nurse*. Brochure. Washington, D.C.: ANA Publishing.

————. 1996a. *Registered Professional Nurses and Unlicensed Assistive Personnel*. 2nd ed. Washington, D.C.: ANA Publishing.

————. 1996b. *Scope and Standards of Advanced Practice Registered Nursing*. Washington, D.C.: ANA Publishing.

American Organization of Nurse Executives. 1996. *Talking Points on Hospital Redesign*. Washington, D.C.: American Organization of Nurse Executives.

Ashton, J., and Fike, R., eds. 1996. *Reengineering for Patient-Focused Care*. Boston: Prescott Publishing.

Bayley, E. et al. 1997. "Preparing to Change from Acute to Community Based Care." *Journal of Nursing Administration* 27:5.

Bernard, L. and Walsh, M. 1996. *Leadership: The Key to Professionalization of Nursing*. New York: Mosby.

Beyers, M. 1996. "The Value of Nursing." *Hospitals and Health Networks*, 5 February, 52.

Chriss, L. 1996. "Nurses Learn How to Work with Assistants." *NurseWeek*, 30 September, 1–3.

Christensen, P., and Bender, L. 1994. "Models of Nursing Care in a Changing Environment." *Orthopaedic Nursing* 13(2): 64–70.

Clarkson Hospital. 1995. "Patient Focused Care." Presentation handouts, June, Omaha, Nebraska.

Coile, R. 1993. "California Hospitals in the 21st Century." *California Hospitals*, November/December, 7–10.

Commonwealth Fund. 1995. *Healthcare Statistics*. Washington, D.C.: US Health Care Financing Administration.

Conti, R. 1996. "Nurse Case Manager Roles: Implications for Practice." *Nursing Administration Quarterly* 21:1.

Curran, C., ed. 1990. "IDN Core Competencies and Nursing's Role." *Nursing Economics*, December.

Davis, C., ed. 1996. *Nursing Staff in Hospitals and Nursing Homes: Is It Adequate?* National Institute of Medicine. Washington, D.C.: National Academy Press.

Dillon, P. 1997. "The Future of Associate Degree Nursing." *Nursing and Healthcare: Perspectives on Community* 18:1.

Donaho, B., ed. 1996. *Celebrating the Journey: A Final Report on Strengthening Hospital Nursing*. Philadelphia: National Academy Press.

Federwisch, A. 1998. "Attitude Matters." *NurseWeek*, 26 January, 13.

Golub, E. 1995. "Revisiting Our Ideas About Health." *Hospitals and Health Networks*, 20 January, 78.

Gray, B.B. 1994a. "Twenty-First Century Hospital Embodies New Concept." *NurseWeek*, 1 April, 1.

————. 1994b. "Changing Skill Mix Reorders Healthcare Delivery System." *NurseWeek*, 2 December, 14.

————. 1995a. "Nurses Face Ethics of Rationing as Healthcare Industry Evolves." *NurseWeek*, 2 April, 20–22.

————. 1995b. "Issues at the Crossroads." Parts 1 and 2. *NurseWeek*, 1 October, 1.

Hagland, M. 1998. "Managing Diseases by Managing IT." *Health Management Technology*, June, 18–25.

Hammers, M.A. 1994. "Crystal Ball Gazing with Leland Kaiser." *RN Times*, 5 September, 8–10.

Harrington, C., and Estes, C., eds. 1997. *Health Policy and Nursing*. 2nd ed. Boston: Jones and Barlett.

Hudson, T. 1997. "Ties That Bind." *Hospitals and Health Networks*, March, 20–26.

Keepnews, D., and Marullo, G. 1996. "Policy Imperatives for Nursing in an Era of Healthcare Restructuring." *Nursing Administration Quarterly* 20(3): 19–31 (spring).

Kunen, J. 1996. "The New Hands-Off Nursing." *Time*, 30 September, 55–57.

Lee, S. 1996. "A Primer on Disease Management." *The Remington Report*, September/October, 30–33.

Manthey, M. 1994. "Issues in Patient Care Delivery." *Journal of Nursing Administration* 24(12): 14–16.

Manuel, P., and Sorensen, L. 1995. "Changing Trends in Healthcare: Implications for Baccalaureate Education, Practice and Employment." *Journal of Nursing Education* 34(6): 248–253.

McCloskey, J., and Grace, H. 1997. *Current Issues in Nursing.* 5th ed. New York: Mosby.

McKinnon, B. 1996. "Is Disease State Management a Strategy for Success or Just Another Industry Buzzword?" *The Remington Report*, September/October, 26–29.

McManis, G.L. 1993. "Reinventing the System." *Hospitals and Health Networks*, 5 October, 42–48.

Merisalo, L., ed. 1998. "Investment in High-Tech Infrastructure Key to Future Success." *Managed Care Payment Advisor*, January, 1–2.

Organization of Nurse Leaders. 1995. "Focus Group Notes." *Nursing Issues.* 29 September.

Pallarito, K. 1996. "Deloitte Survey Identifies Service Consolidation as Key to Efficiency." *Modern Healthcare*, 24 June, 3.

Pew Health Professions Commission. 1995. "Healthy America: Practitioners for 2005." *Pew Health Professions Report.* Washington, D.C.: Pew Health Professions Commission.

———. 1998. *"Pew Health Professions Report.* Washington, D.C.: Pew Health Professions Commission.

Public Policy Institute of California. 1996. *Nursing Staff Trends in California Hospitals: 1977–1995.* October. Sacramento, California: Public Policy Institute of California.

Sampson, E. 1996. "Disease State Management: New Models for Case Management." *The Remington Report*, September/October, 21–25.

Shortell, S. et al. 1996. *Remaking Healthcare in America.* San Francisco: Jossey-Bass.

Simmons, H. 1998. "The Forces That Impact Healthcare-Quality and Costs." *Healthcare Forum Journal*, January/February, 27–46.

Solovy, A. 1998. "Trendspotting." *Hospitals and Health Networks*, 20 March, 60–64.

St. Vincent Hospital. 1994. "CARE 2000: An Approach to Patient Focused Care." Presentation handouts, February.

Sund, J. et al. 1998. "Case Management in an Integrated Delivery System." *Nursing Management*, January, 24–32.

Truscott, J.P., and Churchill, G.M. 1995. "Patient Focused Care." *Nursing Policy Forum* 1(4): 5–12.

Zander, K., ed. 1998. Newsletter. *New Definition* (winter): 1.

# CHAPTER 13

# Nursing for the Future

To utilize your expanding horizons and cope with the changes in your organization, you need to acquire some survival skills. Survival skills for organizational change at work include being perceived as a valuable employee for the organization. Workers who are not perceived as assisting the organization in achieving its objectives are not valuable workers and are at risk for downsizing or role elimination.

It is important to understand the rationale for downsizing of management and workers in your own facility. While you may not agree with the reasons, it is important to the organization that you are perceived as supportive of the changes. Hospitals need help to eliminate fragmentation and departmental barriers. Nurses are in a position to assist facilities in identifying those areas of duplication, fragmentation, and obstruction between departments.

Nurses can support the concept of cross-training. It's no longer a dirty word! Nurses will benefit from the free on-the-job skills training that facilities offer, especially those outside the hospital. Think of all of your skills as a tool kit. Hospitals who cross-train you give you free additions to your tool kit and more to put on your resume. Facilities want to see nurses support safe and quality-based cross-training programs. It is to your personal benefit to do so.

Nurses can also assist facilities by determining ways to move services to the customers and focus more on the total community. Nurses are able to define, develop, and participate in methods to measure care quality as well as physician and customer satisfaction. Working with management to address issues of quality and satisfaction will lead to greater input into changes and more recognition for the key role nurses play in providing health care in all settings.

Hospitals will continue to focus on streamlining processes, systems, and documentation. To assist them, nurses must stay informed about internal and external regulatory health care changes and factors that affect internal processes and systems. Nurses can also offer support by assisting hospitals to facilitate partnering with physicians, either in clinical programs or with contracting entities. It is important for nurses to be aware of what physician contracting entities exist in their facilities, and who are the most significant payers that contract with the hospital.

## CORE COMPETENCIES

Core competencies for RNs of the future include:

1. Critical thinking skills
   - critical decision making
   - strategic, comparative, and contextual thinking
2. Communication skills
   - conflict management
   - delegation and supervision
   - negotiation and assertiveness
   - interpersonal relationship enhancement
3. Leadership skills
   - risk-taking and agency for change
   - role modeling
   - ability to deal with ambiguity
   - flexibility and adaptation
   - teamwork approach
   - problem solving, evaluation, and analysis
   - supervising/overseeing the work of others
4. Collaborative skills
   - advocacy

- partnering with patients, families, and providers in care delivery systems
- multidisciplinary approach
- ability to work with unlicensed assistive personnel and other health care providers
5. Technological skills
   - data management
   - patient care enhancement
   - cross-application of principles
   - efficient substitution for non–patient care functions

## WORKING WITH UNLICENSED ASSISTIVE PERSONNEL

As the acuity of patients and the complexity of their needs have both increased, hospitals and other health care facilities have made major changes in patient care staffing mixes and methods of care delivery. When reengineering was implemented in hospitals a number of years ago, many of them first started by downsizing registered nurse roles and replacing those RNs with unlicensed assistive personnel (UAPs). While numerous hospitals have begun to recognize RN contributions to patient outcomes and have resumed rehiring of professional nurses, the UAP role is likely here to stay.

Unlicensed assistive personnel are defined by the American Nurses' Association as "...individuals who are trained to function in an assistive role to the registered professional nurse in the provision of patient/client care activities as delegated by and under the supervision of the registered professional nurse" (ANA, 1996).

UAPs have been used to provide patient care in different settings for decades. Certified nurses' aides (CNAs) provide the majority of patient care tasks under the direction of a registered nurse in long-term care and skilled nursing facilities. CNAs and UAPs have worked under the direction of professional registered nurses in hospitals, especially in the 1960s and 1970s, in a model then known as "team leading."

Using UAPs as described above enhanced the patient care and allowed the registered nurse to attend to more demanding professional tasks, such as patient assessment, care planning, complex procedures, medication administration, patient education, and evaluation of nursing and medical care outcomes. Registered nurses remained responsible for all aspects of the nursing process for patients.

Within the past decade, reports from registered nurses around the country have indicated increased use of UAPs as *replacements* for registered nurses. Not only have UAPs increased in number, but the kinds of tasks and functions they are called upon to perform have grown in complexity, require significant exercise of judgment, and carry a considerable degree of patient risk (ANA, 1996a).

This is not the intended use—nor a safe use—of UAPs. UAPs do not receive mandatory training; for many UAPs, training is on the job. Critical thinking skills, judgment, and patient assessment are all skills taught at the professional RN level of education. The optimal and cost-effective utilization of UAPs is as assistants to, not replacements for, registered nurses, and the continual clinical oversight of UAPs by the registered professional nurse is essential.

The term UAP encompasses a wide variety of job titles in the hospital setting, including nursing or patient aide, orderly, technician, or attendant. In long-term care settings, the title of nurses' aide is the primary job title because it is defined by federal statue. This is also true of the home health aide in home health care.

The use of UAPs requires training for both the UAP and the RN. The UAP must learn which patient signs and symptoms to report to the registered nurse supervising the patient's care, as well as how to effectively make reports. Professional registered nurses need to learn how to delegate and oversee the work of others. These skills are not usually taught in nursing school. Although many hospitals have reengineered patient care, including the role of UAP, few initiated any training for RN or UAP staff. This is not only frustrating but dangerous for all staff.

The utilization of UAPs has increased dramatically in the past 10 years. Prior to that time, the use of RN staff increased due to rising patient acuity and more sophisticated technology. During the time of increased RN staff usage, the Medicare **prospective payment system** (PPS) was instituted for hospital inpatient services. Hospitals initially attempted to reduce RN staff and increase UAPs, hoping to save money due to Medicare payment limits imposed by PPS. As hospitals increased their reliance on UAPs, limitations of UAPs' abilities and education in the face of complex care became evident. Many institutions found that professional nurses had broad-based skills and abilities that actually made them more cost-effective over time. In fact, some facilities went back to having almost exclusively registered nurses on staff. This is an expensive way to provide patient care.

While the use of UAPs to *replace* registered nurses has proved to be neither risk-free nor cost-effective, there is no reason why UAPs cannot continue to be safely used to *assist* RNs in performing patient care tasks under supervision. The individual professional nurse and the nursing profession have the responsibility of controlling the training, practice, and utilization of UAP roles involved in providing direct patient care.

Health care facilities must base their policies and use of UAPs on demonstrating and ensuring quality patient care. Appropriate roles, skills training, job descriptions, and responsibilities must be developed for use of UAPs and to support the RNs supervising their care.

Registered nurses must be trained to provide supervision and delegation for UAPs. Supervision is the active process of directing, guiding, and influencing the outcome of an individual's performance of an activity. Delegation is described as the transfer of responsibility for the performance of an activity from one individual to another, with the former retaining accountability (ANA, 1996a). Without adequate training and oversight, it is unsafe to have even basic nursing tasks delegated to UAPs. There are other professional nursing tasks, such as assessment, patient teaching, and evaluation of treatment, that should *never* be delegated to UAPs.

Registered nurses can safely use and work with UAPs as long as they follow some important guidelines:

- Keep up with what is happening in health care on both state and national levels.
- Participate in developing and evaluating programs involving delegation of nursing tasks in your own facility.
- Let your nurse manager and hospital administrator know what is and what is not working.
- Support revisions in education for both RNs and UAPs.
- Continue your own professional and personal growth.

When working with UAPs, try to use the following guidelines. They will help you give safe and effective guidance as well as protection for your patients:

- Know your UAPs' qualifications.
- Identify the purpose of the intervention to be delegated.
- Be familiar with your facility's job descriptions and policies.
- Be sure your UAPs have been trained to perform the job duties and tasks assigned to their role.
- Foster communication and trust with UAPs.
- Be specific with your requests.
- Indicate and identify your priorities for patient care.
- Verify UAP understanding and comprehension of the request.
- Double-check your attitude.
- Look for opportunities to teach and explain to UAPs.
- Be aware of the likely results when deciding to delegate.
- Evaluate the potential for harm to the patient.
- Determine the complexity of the task.
- Recognize that problem solving, innovation, evaluation, and adapting activities are registered nursing tasks (AACN, 1996).

Remember that you are all on the same patient care team. The changing health care scenario demands that we no longer put our heads in the sand and ignore the compelling realities before us. We need to assign appropriate nursing tasks to unlicensed assistive personnel. Unlicensed assistive personnel are a valuable resource in today's dynamic health care environment. Recognizing their effectiveness as well as their limitations can benefit everyone—patients, facilities, professional nurses, and UAPs themselves.

## NURSING ROLES OF THE FUTURE

As pointed out so effectively by Ed O'Neil, Executive Director of the Pew Health Professions Commission, nurses have been focusing on the floor of their professional role. They must start focusing on the ceiling because that is where the opportunities are.

Given the trends in health care delivery discussed above, there are numerous role opportunities for RNs. Increasing accountability, management of complex patients, and care delivery will be the foundations of these new roles. Roles for registered nurses exist as advanced practice providers, ambulatory care nurses, physician group practice nurses, parish nurses, industrial/occupational nurses, and as specialized care providers, such as skilled nursing facility and home care nurses.

One of the burgeoning arenas for nurses is home care. Home care of patients has accelerated in the past decade, leaving numerous opportunities for nurses. Ambulatory care is another fast-growing segment of nursing. Physician group practices, clinics, schools, churches, IPAs, and disease management programs are all facilities where nurses can find unparalleled opportunities.

Nurse entrepreneurs can find new career options. All types of consulting, private practice, and group practices are new models for nursing practice. Advanced practice nurses such as nurse practitioners, midwives, and anesthetists are setting up group practices successfully. Self-direction, setting your own work schedule, and choosing whom you work with are benefits of entrepreneurship. Being your own boss is highly rewarding. Reimbursement regulations are continuing to change to allow advanced practice nurses direct reimbursement.

Another fast-growing area of nursing is nursing informatics. Nurses blend their knowledge of nursing practice with information technology to design and direct health care delivery information technology and practice. This is a dynamic role for nurses.

As nurses stop "protecting the floor" and start "reaching for the ceiling," their opportunities and options will be unprecedented. Start evaluating what you need to do to get ready for the future!

---

There are many opportunities for nurses in the future. Preparing for these new and changing roles include many of the concepts from this book:
- career management strategies
- interpersonal skills
- basic business skills
- computer literacy
- higher education (baccalaureate level minimum)
- focus practice outside the hospital

## DISCUSSION QUESTIONS

1. What are the most important nursing skills for the future for nurses in your geographic area? Why?
2. Are nurses currently taught skills important to their future roles in your geographic area? Why or why not?
3. List five skills for the future that are important to your nursing role.
4. List four roles that you would enjoy in the future.
5. Are UAPs used in your facility? For what tasks?
6. What type of training was provided for UAPs at your facility or in your local geographic area?
7. What types of care are UAPs currently providing that may be unsafe or inappropriate? Why?

---

### BIBLIOGRAPHY

Aiken, L. et al. 1994. "Lower Medicare Mortality among a Set of Hospitals Known for Good Nursing Care." *Medical Care* 32(8), June, 771–785.

American Academy of Nursing. Goertzen, I., ed. 1990. "Differentiated Nursing Practice into the Twenty-First Century." *Selected Papers from The American Academy of Nursing. Washington, D.C.: ANA Publishing.*

American Association of Ambulatory Care Nurses. 1996. *Standards for Ambulatory Care Nursing.* Aliso Viejo, California: AACN.

American Association of Colleges of Nursing. 1995. *Essentials of Masters Education for Advanced Practice Nursing.* Unpublished.

American Association of Colleges of Nursing, American Organization of Nurse Executives, and National Organization for Associate Degree Nursing. 1995. *A Model for Differentiated Nursing Practice.* Washington, D.C.: AACN.

American Association of Critical-Care Nurses. 1996. "Decision Grid for Delegation." Staffing Tool Kit. Washington, D.C.: AACN Publishing.

American Nurses' Association. 1985. *Code for Nurses.* Washington, D.C.: ANA Publishing.

———. 1993. *Nursing's Agenda for Health Care Reform.* Washington, D.C.: ANA Publishing.

———. 1994. *Every Patient Deserves a Nurse.* Brochure. Washington, D.C.: ANA Publishing.

———. 1995. *Nursing's Social Policy Statement.* Washington, D.C.: ANA Publishing.

———. 1996a. *Registered Professional Nurses and Unlicensed Assistive Personnel.* 2nd ed. Washington, D.C.: ANA Publishing.

————. 1996b. *Scope and Standards of Advanced Practice Registered Nursing.* Washington, D.C.: ANA Publishing.

American Organization of Nurse Executives. 1996. *Talking Points on Hospital Redesign.* Washington, D.C.: American Organization of Nurse Executives.

Ashton, J., and Fike, R., eds. 1996. *Reengineering for Patient-Focused Care.* Boston: Prescott Publishing.

Bayley, E. et al. 1997. "Preparing to Change from Acute to Community Based Care." *Journal of Nursing Administration* 27:5.

Beakley, P. 1998. "Are You Smart Enough for Your Job?" *University of Phoenix* (spring): 14–16.

Beckham, J.D. 1997a. "The Right Way to Integrate." *Healthcare Forum Journal,* July/August, 30–37.

————. 1997b. "The Beginning of the End for HMOs." Part 1. *Healthcare Forum Journal,* November/December, 44–47.

————. 1998. "The Beginning of the End for HMOs." Part 2. *Healthcare Forum Journal,* January/February, 52–55.

Bergman, R. 1993. "Quantum Leaps." *Hospitals and Health Networks,* 5 October, 28–35.

————. 1994. "Reengineering Health Care." *Hospitals and Health Networks,* 5 February, 16–24.

Bernard, L., and Walsh, M. 1996. *Leadership: The Key to Professionalization of Nursing.* New York: Mosby.

Beyers, M. 1996. "The Value of Nursing." *Hospitals and Health Networks,* 5 February, 52.

Brink, S. et al. 1997. "America's Top HMOs." *US News and World Report,* 13 October, 60–69.

Brock, R. 1996. "Head for Business." *Hospitals and Health Networks,* 5 December, 62–66.

Burda, D. 1994a. "A Profit by Any Other Name Would Still Give Hospitals the Fits." *Modern Healthcare,* 8 August, 115–136.

————. 1994b. "Layoffs Rise as Pace of Cost-Cutting Accelerates." *Modern Healthcare,* 12 December, 32.

————. 1995. "ANA Report Stokes Restructuring Debate." *Modern Healthcare,* 13 February, 38.

Burns, J. 1993. "Caring for the Community." *Modern Healthcare,* 8 November, 30–33.

Butts, J., and Brock, A. 1996. "Optimizing Nursing through Reorganization: Mandates for the New Millennium." *Nursing Connections* 9(4): 49–58.

California Strategic Planning Committee for Nursing. 1996. *Final Report.* Irvine, California: California Strategic Planning Committee for Nursing.

Christensen, P., and Bender, L. 1994. "Models of Nursing Care in a Changing Environment." *Orthopaedic Nursing* 13(2): 64–70.

Clarkson Hospital. 1995. "Patient Focused Care." Presentation handouts, June, Omaha, Nebraska.

Coile, R. 1993a. "California Healthcare 2001: The Outlook for America's Bellwether State." *Hospital Strategy Report* 5(4), February.

———. 1993b. "California Hospitals in the 21st Century." *California Hospitals*, November/December, 7–10.

———. 1994a. "Primary Care Networks: The Integrators of Care in an Integrated Delivery System." *Hospital Strategy Report* 6(8): 1–3.

———. 1994b. "Capitation: The New Food Chain of HMO Provider Payment." *Hospital Strategy Report* 6(9): 1–3.

Conti, R. 1996. "Nurse Case Manager Roles: Implications for Practice." *Nursing Administration Quarterly* 21:1.

Curran, C., ed. 1990. "IDN Core Competencies and Nursing's Role." *Nursing Economics*, December.

Davis, C., ed. 1996. *Nursing Staff in Hospitals and Nursing Homes: Is It Adequate?* National Institute of Medicine. Washington, D.C.: National Academy Press.

Dillon, P. 1997. "The Future of Associate Degree Nursing." *Nursing and Healthcare: Perspectives on Community* 18:1.

Donaho, B., ed. 1996. *Celebrating the Journey: A Final Report on Strengthening Hospital Nursing*. Philadelphia: National Academy Press.

Dracup, K., and Bryan-Brown, C., eds. 1998. "Thinking Outside the Box and Other Resolutions." *American Journal of Critical-Care*, January, 1.

Eck, S. et al. 1997. "Consumerism, Nursing and the Reality of Resources." *Nursing Administration Quarterly* 12(3): 1–11.

Flower, J. 1997a. "Job Shift." *Healthcare Forum Journal*, January/February, 15–24.

———. 1997b. "The Age of Heretics." *Healthcare Forum Journal*, March/April, 34–39.

Golub, E. 1995. "Revisiting Our Ideas about Health." *Hospitals and Health Networks*, 20 January, 78.

Goodman, J. 1993. "Twenty Myths about National Health Insurance." Dallas, Tex.: National Center for Policy Analysis.

Gray, B.B. 1994a. "Twenty-First Century Hospital Embodies New Concept." *NurseWeek*, 1 April, 1.

———. 1994b. "Changing Skill Mix Reorders Healthcare Delivery System." *NurseWeek*, 2 December, 14.

———. 1995a. "Nurses Face Ethics of Rationing as Healthcare Industry Evolves." *NurseWeek*, 2 April, 20–22.

———. 1995b. "Issues at the Crossroads." Parts 1 and 2. *NurseWeek*, 1 October, 1.

Grayson, M., ed. 1995. "Clinical Maneuvers." *Hospitals and Health Networks*, 5 January, 52.

———. 1997. "Stuck on a Strategy." *Hospitals and Health Networks*, 5 October, 74–76.

———. 1998. "Back to the Future." *Hospitals and Health Networks*, 20 January, 7.

Grimaldi, P. 1998. "PSO Requirements Taking Shape." *Nursing Management*, February, 14–18.

Groves, M. 1996. "Life After Layoffs." *Los Angeles Times*, 25 March, 3.

Hagland, M. 1995. "Incent Me." *Hospitals and Health Networks*, 5 September, 7.

Hammer, M., and Champy, S. 1995. *Reengineering the Corporation*. New York: Harper Collins.

Hammers, M.A. 1994. "Crystal Ball Gazing with Leland Kaiser." *RN Times*, 5 September, 8–10.

Healthcare Advisory Board. 1992a. "Executive Report to the CEO: The Merits of Patient-Focused Care." Acetate presentation, October, The Advisory Board Company, Washington, D.C.

———. 1992b. "Toward a Twenty-First Century Hospital: Designing Patient Care." Acetate presentation, October, The Advisory Board Company, Washington, D.C.

Hirsch, G. 1997. "Fit to Be Tried." *Hospitals and Health Networks*, 5 November, 50–54.

Hudson, T. 1997. "Ties That Bind." *Hospitals and Health Networks*, March, 20–26.

Izzo, J. 1998. "The Changing Values of Workers." *Healthcare Forum Journal*, May/June, 62–65.

Keepnews, D., and Marullo, G. 1996. "Policy Imperatives for Nursing in an Era of Healthcare Restructuring." *Nursing Administration Quarterly* 20(3): 19–31 (spring).

Kemp, V.H. 1995. "Overview of Change and Leadership." *Contemporary Leadership Behavior*. 2nd ed. Boston: Little Brown and Company, 275–282.

Kertesz, L. 1997. "What's Right, Wrong?" *Modern Healthcare*, 11 August, 70–74.

Koerner, J.G., and Karpiuk, K.L. 1994. *Implementing Differentiated Nursing Practice: Transformation by Design*. Gaithersburg, MD: Aspen Publishers, Inc.

Kunen, J. 1996. "The New Hands-Off Nursing." *Time*, 30 September, 55–57.

Lanara, V.A. 1993. "The Nurse of the Future, Role and Function." *Journal of Nursing Management* 1: 83–87.

Lee, S. 1996. "A Primer on Disease Management." *The Remington Report*, September/October, 30–33.

Lumsdon, K. 1994a. "It's a Jungle Out There!" *Hospitals and Health Networks*, 20 May, 68–72.

———. 1994b. "Want to Save Millions?" *Hospitals and Health Networks*, 5 November, 24–32.

———. 1995a. "Watch for Flying Phrases." *Hospitals and Health Networks*, 20 March, 79–81.

———. 1995b. "Mean Streets." *Hospitals and Health Networks*, 5 October, 44–52.

———. 1995c. "Working Smarter, Not Harder." *Hospitals and Health Networks*, 5 November, 27–31.

———. 1995d. "Faded Glory." *Hospitals and Health Networks*, 5 December, 31–36.

MacStravic, S. 1988. "Outcome Marketing in Healthcare." *Healthcare Management Review* 13(2): 53–59.

———. 1997. "Managing Demand: The Wrong Paradigm." *Managed Care Quarterly* 5(4): 8–17.

Malone, B. et al. 1996. "A Grim Prognosis for Healthcare." *American Journal of Nursing Survey Results*, November, 40.

Manion, J. 1996. "Understanding the Seven Stages of Change." *RN Magazine*, April, 21.

Manthey, M. 1994. "Issues in Patient Care Delivery." *Journal of Nursing Administration* 24(12): 14–16.

Manuel, P., and Sorensen, L. 1995. "Changing Trends in Healthcare: Implications for Baccalaureate Education, Practice and Employment." *Journal of Nursing Education* 34(6): 248–253.

Marks, M. 1994. *From Turmoil to Triumph*. New York: Lexington Press.

McCloskey, J., and Grace, H. 1997. *Current Issues in Nursing*. 5th ed. New York: Mosby.

McManis, G.L. 1993. "Reinventing the System." *Hospitals and Health Networks*, 5 October, 42–48.

Merisalo, L., ed. 1998a. "Investment in High-Tech Infrastructure Key to Future Success." *Managed Care Payment Advisor*, January, 1–2.

———., ed. 1998b. "RN Staff Cuts Due to Managed Care Pressures May Be Costly." *Managed Care Payment Advisor*, March, 1–2.

Miller, J. 1995. "Leading Nursing into the Future." *Harvard Nursing Research Institute Newsletter* 4(3): 5–7.

Moore, J.D., Jr. 1998. "What Downsizing." *Modern Healthcare*, 19 January, 12.

Morrell, J. 1995. "Turn Your Focus Outside In." *Hospitals and Health Networks*, 5 December, 66.

Organization of Nurse Leaders. 1995. "Focus Group Notes." *Nursing Issues.* 29 September.

O'Rourke, M.W. 1996. "Who Holds the Keys to the Future of Healthcare?" *NurseWeek*, 8 January, 1.

Pallarito, K. 1996. "Deloitte Survey Identifies Service Consolidation as Key to Efficiency." *Modern Healthcare*, 24 June, 3.

Pew Health Professions Commission. 1995. "Healthy America: Practitioners for 2005." *Pew Health Professions Report*. Washington, D.C.: Pew Health Professions Commission.

———. 1998. *Pew Health Professions Report*. Washington, D.C.: Pew Health Professions Commission.

Pinto, C. et al. 1998. "Future Trends." *Modern Healthcare*, 5 January, 27–40.

Porter-O'Grady, T. 1994. "Working with Consultants on a Redesign." *American Journal of Nursing,* October, 33–39.

Public Policy Institute of California. 1996. *Nursing Staff Trends in California Hospitals: 1977–1995.* October. Sacramento, California: Public Policy Institute of California.

Rich, P.L. 1995. "Working with Nursing Assistants: Becoming a Team." *Nursing 95*, May, 100–103.

RN Scope of Practice. California Business and Professions Code, sec. 2725.

RN Special Advisory Committee. 1990. *Meeting the Immediate and Future Needs for Nursing in California*. Sacramento, California: State of California.

Sampson, E. 1996. "Disease State Management: New Models for Case Management." *The Remington Report*, September/October, 21-25.

Sheehy, B. et al., 1995. "Don't Blink or You'll Miss It." *The Atlanta Consulting Group*, Atlanta, 69–87.

Sherer, J. 1994a. "Corporate Cultures." *Hospitals and Health Networks*, 5 May, 20–27.

———. 1994b. "Job Shifts." *Hospitals and Health Networks*, 5 October, 64–68.

———. 1995. "Tapping into Teams." *Hospitals and Health Networks*, 5 July, 32–35.

Shindul-Rothschild, J. et al. 1997. "Ten Keys to Quality Care." *American Journal of Nursing* 97(11): 35–43.

Shortell, S. et al. 1996. *Remaking Healthcare in America*. San Francisco: Jossey-Bass.

Shubert, D. 1996. "Hospitals Decrease Nurses' Role: Reassign Tasks to Aides." *Los Angeles Times*, 14 July.

Simmons, H. 1998. "The Forces That Impact Healthcare—Quality and Costs." *Healthcare Forum Journal*, January/February, 27–46.

Stewart, T. 1993. "Reengineering: The Hot New Management Tool." *Fortune*, 23 August, 41–45.

St. Vincent Hospital. 1994. "CARE 2000: An Approach to Patient Focused Care." Presentation handouts, February 1994.

Sund, J. et al. 1998. "Case Management in an Integrated Delivery System." *Nursing Management*, January, 24–32.

Truscott, J.P., and Churchill, G.M. 1995. "Patient Focused Care." *Nursing Policy Forum* 1(4): 5–12.

Turner, S.O. 1995a. "Stand Out or Lose Out." *Nursing 95*, January, 13–18.

———. 1995b. "Managing Your Transition: Strategies for the Future." *Surgical Services Management*, May, 40–42.

———. 1995c. "Reality Check: It's Time for Nursing to Face the Future." *Hospitals and Health Networks*, 20 August, 20–22.

———. 1995d. "Nurses: Are They the Key to Successful Capitation?" *Capitation and Medical Practice*, December, 1–2.

———. 1996. "Capitation: Are You Ready for It?" *Surgical Services Management*, February, 43–45.

Ummel, S. 1997. "Integration." *Healthcare Forum Journal*, March/April, 13–27.

Van, S. 1994. "A New Attitude." *RN Times*, November, 12–13.

Wesorick, B. "Standards: On the Cutting Edge or Over the Cliff?" *Notes on Clinical Practice, 1990s*. Unpublished paper.

Zander, K., ed. 1998. Newsletter. *New Definition* (winter), 1.

# CHAPTER 14

# Career Issues for Nurses in a Managed Care Delivery System

Stress is unavoidable. It is a natural reaction to changes in your life—pleasant as well as unpleasant changes. When you feel anxious or excited, your body turns on the "fight-or-flight" mechanism that revs you up to cope with a challenge. The physiological response is the same whether you are fleeing from a mugger or beating a close deadline.

## STRESS AND NURSES IN TODAY'S HEALTH CARE ENVIRONMENT

When channeled constructively, the surge of energy, concentration, and power triggered by the stress alarm can spur you on to greater productivity and creativity. When stress is unrelenting, this energy-draining mobilization can lead to health problems ranging from headaches to heart attacks.

Nurses are no strangers to stress. Because of changes in the health care environment, nurses in all roles in any facility face more stress than ever before. Researchers have come to believe that there are three kinds of stress: normal, good, and bad. Each type of stress has a different effect on the body. Normal stress keeps you on your toes when circumstances call for action. Good stress mobilizes and galvanizes you with raring-to-go excitement and enthusiasm. Bad stress is chronic stress that causes the fight-or-flight response to kick in habitually to the point of wearing out the body.

167

The fight-or-flight response primes you to deal with a threat physically. Stress hormones, including adrenaline, flood into your bloodstream, causing your breathing to quicken, your heart to race, and oxygen-rich blood to concentrate in your brain and muscles for quick action.

In today's challenging and difficult health care environment, you are more likely to face an emotional or mental challenge than a life-or-death threat. When your body cannot act on a stress signal, there is no physical quick release for the potent chemicals circulating through your bloodstream. Normally, once a perceived threat is over, your body gradually brings itself back into balance. Heart rate, metabolism, and breathing slow down. However, if stress continues without a break for long periods of time, you never have a chance to recover. Over time, elevated heartbeat leads to high blood pressure, and stress hormones build up in the blood to damage vessels and arteries.

People vary in the type and amount of pressure they can tolerate, but ultimately the body has a limited ability to withstand stress. Stress-related illnesses account for over 75 percent of all visits to physicians. That is why it is important to handle stress before it leads to medical problems.

Two management consultants, Peter McLaughlin and Peter McLaughlin, Jr., determined that there are seven steps to achieving top performance and being your best. They believe that the key to thriving in the tumultuous conditions of today's business climate (which certainly describes health care) is the ability to manage your energy and emotions (1998). Chapter 17, Thriving in the New Environment, will help you understand how to use intuitive skills that many nurses already have. Consider these seven ideas as forming a method to impact your performance by increasing your enthusiasm and focus:

1. Master your mind by staying in tune with your emotional state and energy levels. Self-awareness is vital to consistent excellent performance.
2. Eat for performance and upgrade your eating habits. A good diet provides your body and brain with fuel to run efficiently.
3. Increase exercise to provide gains in energy, confidence, emotional control, and mental clarity.
4. Break up stress and fatigue by re-orchestrating your daily schedule. Plan breaks to relax your mind and refresh your energy.
5. Learn to love problems and see them as challenges.

There is no all-purpose solution for stress and no gauge to measure one's capacity to endure it. The intensity of stress differs for everyone. What is stressful for some people barely ruffles others. But there are effective strategies for relieving tension and coping with problems and pressures:

1. Perform regular aerobic exercise.
2. Adjust your own perceptions so that you are actually evaluating *situations*, not just your *perceptions* about the situations.
3. Nurture a sense of being in control instead of powerlessness.
4. Adjust your attitude from a negative and reactive to a positive and proactive approach.
5. Take charge of your life by maintaining your sense of purpose and focus.
6. Be open to change.
7. See changes as challenges, not threats.
8. Visualize success.
9. Control and manage your time.
10. Learn to let go of what doesn't matter.
11. Plan time to relax and have fun.
12. Save time for yourself.

6. Put your humor to work. Humor can help you tolerate the ambiguity of health care as well as assist you in remaining poised in impossible situations.
7. Create an energizing environment—enhance your physical workplace with personal inspiration (McLaughlin and McLaughlin, 1998).

## COPING WITH DOWNSIZING

I became an entrepreneur and a self-employed consultant after receiving three layoffs in five years—before it was trendy! With all the changes in hospitals and in the health care industry overall, it is unreasonable to think that you might not be affected by downsizing.

It's called many different things . . . downsizing, rightsizing, reduction in force, layoffs. . . . No matter what you call it, it is difficult to deal with.

The scenario usually goes something like this. You have just been called into your nurse-manager's office. She asks you to sit down. She seems uneasy as she remarks on how quickly health care is changing. Eventually, she gets to her point: Your position has been eliminated; you are being laid off (Turner, 1995c).

No matter how it is presented, being laid off always comes as a blow. As a layoff veteran myself, I know just how bad it feels. And although no one can make it all go away, you can at least get what you deserve. By remembering the following tips, you can ensure that you get maximum severance pay and benefits, as well as favorable references from your employer.

Don't panic. Take a deep breath. You will live through this. Don't take it personally. You are not alone. Many good, competent, and long-term employees are being laid off as more and more hospitals restructure. When I speak around the country to nursing conferences and ask how many attendees have been laid off, at least half of every audience raises their hands. It is common to be downsized out of a role these days.

Don't lash out. Getting angry at your manager or senior administrators may reduce your negotiating power for severance pay later. So grit your teeth, don't bad-mouth anyone, and try to appear gracious. Don't try to get even. Nursing is a very incestuous profession where everyone knows everyone. You could be sorry later if you burn your bridges now.

I don't recommend staying in the facility any longer than is absolutely necessary. It breeds frustration, and you feel like a lame duck (which you are). Clear out your locker or office the day you get your notice and turn in your key and name tag. Be sure to take any personal files and items with you. You won't want to come back and pick them up later—it will be too painful. Don't take any hospital property, delete important computer documents, or otherwise undermine projects. Those tactics will harm your ability to get good references later on and could lead to legal action against you.

Try not to discuss severance at that first notification meeting if you can avoid it. Tell your nurse-manager that you are not prepared to discuss the details now, but that you want to make an appointment for a day or two later after you have had time to deal with your emotions and think things through. That way you will negotiate with a clear head.

Document as much as you can about the initial meeting. If possible, take notes during this meeting. Include what each of you said about the layoff. If you are unable to take notes during the meeting, go back to your office or unit and write down as much as you can remember about the meeting. These notes may be useful later.

After you have received your layoff/reduction in force notification, make an appointment with someone in the human resources department. Sometimes human resources staff will come to the initial layoff notification meeting. If so, you can ask questions then. If a representative from human resources is not present during the initial notification meeting, you will need to speak with one separately.

You need to set up a meeting to review your current benefit status. Ask about unpaid sick and vacation time, as well as any language about layoffs in your contract if you are in a unionized facility. If you are enrolled in a retirement or profit-sharing plan, ask about rollovers and buyouts. If you have medical insurance benefits, get all the forms and information about Consolidated Omnibus Budget Reconciliation Act (**COBRA**) health benefits. These are legislated benefits that give you the right to remain insured (at your own expense) for up to 18 months after you are laid off.

Find out if you are eligible for outplacement assistance. This benefit is frequently offered to nurse-managers and middle managers. Sometimes, this benefit can be traded for a lower severance pay package. Outplacement personnel are specially trained staff that assist you with job hunting, creating or updating resumes, creating cover letters, networking with other nurses, learning interviewing techniques, and other skills. This kind of assistance is invaluable to nurses, especially those who have never received formal job counseling. Outplacement experts help you determine what type of job is best for you, help you find job contacts, and give moral support during this difficult time. Outplacement assistance can be a useful negotiating point in lieu of severance pay. So ask about it early in the process and then again later, if you cannot get the severance money you want. Outplacement assistance has cash value and worth, so don't disregard it as a "non-monetary" benefit you don't really need—because you do need it.

Try to remember to ask about references. Find out from your nurse-manager and the human resources representative exactly who will provide your reference information and what will be said. Make any requests for written or verbal references during the discussion about severance pay.

Negotiate hard for severance pay. The rule of thumb is one week per year of service. But most managers feel guilty about layoffs, so use that to your advantage. Ask for twice as much as you think you can get. You can always back down, but you can't negotiate up. If you can't get as many weeks as you deserve, ask for additional vacation or sick-time payout, outplacement services, or job counseling. Any accrued unused sick time and vacation time is usually paid out at the time of layoff. You may be able to negotiate having the time paid out over several pay periods, which will add time to your severance pay. This option varies within organizations.

Apply for unemployment benefits as soon as possible. While it is tempting to delay going to the unemployment office, most unemployment procedures are drawn out. So, the sooner you apply, the sooner your claim will be processed and the sooner you will begin receiving checks. Unemployment procedures vary among states and counties, so check with your local unemployment office for the specific process.

Try to get the word out about your layoff. While this sounds difficult, tell all of your colleagues that you are looking for a job. Be sure they know what kind of position you are interested in. Get their phone numbers and addresses and touch base every now and then. You never know what leads you will turn up. Also inform members of any professional association you belong to. Some associations have set up free job counseling, job banks, and recruitment hot line services. Make sure you know what is available for the asking.

You will need to update or write your resume. By having your resume up-to-date and ready to go, you can jump on any job openings that come along. You will also be able to pass out copies to colleagues who might have leads. You should also have business cards printed. They can simply have your name, address, and phone number. They can be printed very inexpensively at office supply stores, or you can print them on your computer. If you have business cards, people will know how to find you if they have a job or hear of one you might be interested in.

Compile a list of references. First get permission from each person to use him or her as a reference. Include the person's name, title, institution, credentials, address, and phone number. Submit this separate, typed list to prospective employers only if asked.

You may need to brush up on your job-hunting skills. Go to your public library and review books and articles on interviewing and job hunting. In fact, if you have the opportunity, attend an occasional interview while you are employed just to keep your skills up. It may sound like heresy, but these days it's best to stay in practice.

When I was happily ensconced in my nursing role, I declined to interview for any job opportunities that came my way. I did that for eight years—foolishly, as it turned out. When I was laid off—much to my surprise and chagrin—I had no network to contact. All of the recruiters had taken me off their lists and my colleagues all thought I was happy as a clam and didn't need to hear about job opportunities. I had to start over and create my job network from scratch. Don't make the same mistake!

During the highly stressful time after a layoff, take good care of yourself. Get plenty of sleep, eat healthfully, and try to get some exercise. Exercise is a great stress reliever and helps you clear your head. Work on projects around the house you have been putting off. Try to take advantage of the one thing you now have plenty of: time.

Get support. Remember that who you are is not what you do. Be open to receiving support and empathy from family and friends. Talk about your grief, anger, and sense of betrayal with trusted confidants. Seek professional counseling if necessary. It may be tempting to stay in constant contact with employees from the facility you just left. For some individuals, this is comforting. For others, like myself, it was too painful to hear what was going on without being part of it.

Try to give yourself some time off. Take a few days or a week to regroup before you begin job hunting. Reacting to a layoff takes time and so does recovery from one. Be choosy about roles you interview for. Don't take the first job you find. Do a self-assessment about your life, the type of job you are looking for, and your personal short- and long-term career goals. Try to find a job that fits into your life, not one in which your life has to be fitted. If you choose wisely and give yourself some time to adjust, a layoff can turn out to be a blessing in disguise. I know—they were for me!

## SPECIALTY CERTIFICATION: DO YOU NEED IT?

Nursing certification examinations are designed to answer the question of what qualifications nurses really need in order to practice effectively in a specialty area. By definition, certification exams provide standards set by an outside agency for validating an individual nurse's qualifications and knowledge in a particular clinical or functions area. According to Melissa Biel, Director of Certification for the American Association of Critical Care Nurses Certification Corporation, a subsidiary of the American Association of Critical-Care Nurses (AACN), "Certification has the goal of providing consumer protection by validating nurses' knowledge, but certification does not prove knowledge is applied." (personal communication, 1995).

In addition, recognition for certification varies. Marie Reed, director of the American Nurses Credentialing Center (ANCC), a subsidiary of the American Nurses Association (ANA), has said "The issue is that there has not been a lot of research done in the area of certification to indicate that 'yes' it makes a difference. (Reed, 1995)" However, informal recognition exists. Nurse administrators have built certification into their career programs and consideration for job opportunities and promotions. There is also personal, professional, and peer recognition, but it varies from area to area.

Another critical factor is experience. Biel says, "I have to believe that the more experience you have, the better it is for the patient" (personal communication, 1995). Consequently, AACN, ANCC, and other certifying bodies almost always demand a certain amount of academic training through continuing education as well as clinical experience, RN licensure, peer recommendations, and other demonstrations of competence before an applicant is permitted to take a certification examination.

Today, licensed RNs can become certified in more that 30 separate specialties through examination. The ANA Credentialing Center administers 23 such examinations, and other nursing specialty organizations administer the rest. On the whole, the examinations and preparation for them require nurses and often their employers to invest significant amounts of time and resources in the certification process. Fees range from $175 to $300 for certification exams. What exactly does this investment of time and money buy?

Test development represents a lengthy and laborious process. While there are many variations, AACN and ANCC both follow a typical pattern. Experienced nurses in the field submit questions they believe a successful practitioner must be able to answer in order to perform that role in a nursing specialty. In addition, surveys on role definition help test developers in each specialty identify the actual tasks a nurse performs. Taken together, this information becomes the basis for test questions that are then evaluated and revised by a test committee. Once a question is perfected, it is field-tested in an examination setting. Test developers track how well test-takers perform on the question before it becomes a permanent part of a certification examination.

When a nurse meets all of the specialty examination prerequisites and passes the examination, certification is awarded, usually for a specified period of time. Some individuals, like Rita Aumen of the American Board of Post Anesthesia Nursing Certification, believe that the certification process "offers consumer protection, enhances patient care, promotes professionalism, and helps employers identify capable people" (Van, 1994). ANCC's Reed believes that certification is a way for nurses to achieve a broader range of job opportunities, receive bonus pay, and, in some specialties, become eligible for third-party reimbursement.

Not everyone agrees with the benefits of certification. A looming issue concerns certification examination prerequisites. In 1998, both AACN and ANCC require certification examinees to have baccalaureate degrees. Representatives for most nursing specialty organizations say that enhanced prerequisites for certification are not intended to exclude those nurses who do not have baccalaureate degrees. They state that nurses with current licensure will be "grandfathered in" through special provisions when the new prerequisites take effect. Others refer to programs that will assist non-degreed nurses in obtaining further education, allowing them to meet the prerequisites for certification.

There is clearly a trend in nursing toward enhanced preparation, and certification is one method of providing that. The number of nurses taking certification examinations grows by 10 percent each year. Most of the stimulus comes from a concern within nursing about professionalism, recognition, and clout. Because nursing has so many specialties, so many inconsistent certification requirements, and so many modes of entry, by increasing preparations and standardizing certification requirements, nurses could become more politically empowered.

Consistent quality of service is a particularly important issue in the profession. Margretta Styles, who authored the ANA's 1988 report *"On Specialization in Nursing: Toward a New Empowerment,"* says, "[S]pecialties wishing to be recognized must strive to achieve the standards set by the profession and the most respected specialties. Indices of quality are educational standards, practice standards, certification and accreditation standards and research productivity and dissemination. A specialty of lesser standards should anticipate a tenuous future within a fluctuating system" (Van, 1994). Styles's prescriptions may seem remote from day-to-day nursing practice; many feel that more rigorous standards are likely to be a hallmark of future certification examinations. This trend is strengthened by the expectation that health care reform may allow advanced specialty and practice nurses to provide a greater range of basic health care services for which they could receive third-party reimbursement, a move that would at the same time reduce the cost of delivering health care services to under-served groups.

As the field of nursing becomes more demanding and complex, the importance of nursing specialty certification will increase. In addition to be-

---

When evaluating certification, consider the following issues and questions:

- Carefully evaluate the exam. Just because it's offered doesn't mean it is valid and reliable.
- Determine that certification will provide you with reimbursement and promotion. Verify this by looking carefully at the issues raised by the application forms for certification examinations.
- How rigorous are the educational requirements?
- What are the clinical practice requirements?
- How carefully are the functions of the nursing specialty worked out?
- Is the content required for the examination indicated, knowledge-tested, and appropriate?
- What is the content based on?
- Is the examination offered by a respected organization that has no possibility of conflicts of interest?
- Check to be sure that the examination addresses nursing standards of practice for that specialty.
- Learn about the organization that gives the certification examination in the specialty area.
- Determine whether specialists in practice in that area determine the content of the exam.
- Validate that the organization offering the examination has met ANA standards for certification.
- Determine if the examination is recognized by the nursing and non-nursing community for its professional standards.
- Be sure the continuing education program is accredited.

ing practitioners, nurses are also consumers. Until certification and ac-creditation are fully established and nationally standardized, certification exams are probably a case in which the warning of "let the buyer beware" may apply.

## NURSING EDUCATION: HOW MUCH IS ENOUGH?

In a recent nursing journal editorial, the Editor-in-Chief of *NurseWeek* magazine suggested that registered nurses needed a bachelor's degree to be considered credible (Gray, March 23, 1998, p. 4). That editorial generated the most reader response from nurses in the history of the magazine.

It begs the obvious question. Does a registered nurse really need a bachelor's degree? The concept of differentiated practice, discussed in Chapter 11 of this book, talks about nursing practice based on both competency *and* education. The criteria for differentiated practice is based on competencies, driven by individual nurse performance as well as nursing school curricula.

How much education do nurses need to do their job? Nurses have been deeply and emotionally divided on this issue for years. There are those who believe that a bachelor's degree should be the minimum educational requirement for a registered professional nurse. Then there are those who believe that the sheer volume of community college and diploma graduates shows that those programs are successful and appropriate.

Barbara Bronson Gray, MN, RN, Editor-in-Chief of *NurseWeek*, argues that nurses are one of the least educated health care professions around (Gray, March 23, 1998). She believes that if patients knew that nurses have less education than most other health care professionals, they would not lobby to have more nurses involved in patient care.

Whether nurses agree or not, a four-year college education is the dividing line for all other professions. If nurses want to sit at the table and negotiate for how dollars are spent on nursing care and coordinate the entire spectrum of care for patients, we have to be educationally on par with other decision makers. As Gray states, college doesn't make a great nurse or physical therapist or teacher or engineer (Gray, March 23, 1998). But what it does do is give you confidence and parity with others in your circle. College also gives you a broader perspective about life and the world.

What holds nurses back in today's health care environment isn't managed care or restructuring or nursing shortages. It's our own unwillingness to bite the bullet and demand more of ourselves. We are poor conflict managers and unable to deal with the unhappiness that such a professional edict would create for some nurses. We shudder at the idea of actually mandating colleagues to do something that will benefit all of us.

While we sit on the sidelines unable to do battle, the health care future and our role in it is being planned around us. We need to proactively determine our professional destiny—or someone else will do it for us. If we don't make a college degree mandatory, Gray says we can forget the questions of prestige, power, and salary (Gray, March 23, 1998). True, but what educational parity is really about is pride, accountability, and accepting that if we want to play with the "big boys" we have to be seen as part of the health care team. Being on the team means getting a vote and getting a vote means helping our patients—the reason most of us became nurses in the first place!

## DISCUSSION QUESTIONS

1. Identify five behaviors you have seen exhibited by health care providers that may indicate stress.
2. List four behaviors you have exhibited that are indicative of stress.
3. Can stress be prevented? Should it be? Why or why not?
4. How can nurses proactively handle stress in their roles? Explain.
5. Are nurses in your geographic location being laid off or downsized? Hired? Why or why not?
6. Are nurses in your geographic location coping effectively with downsizing or layoffs? Why or why not?
7. What are the union activities for unions who represent nurses in your geographic area? Are those activities proactive? reactive? Why? Are the activities related or unrelated to downsizing or layoffs?
8. Should there be a mandatory entry level of education for nurses at the baccalaureate level? Why or why not?
9. What are the most important qualities or characteristics provided to nurses during their education?
10. Should health care providers require specific education for specific roles? Why or why not?

## BIBLIOGRAPHY

Adizes, S. 1993. *Mastering Change*. Pacific Palisades, California: Adizes Institute Publications.

Austin, N. 1995. "The Skill Every Manager Must Master." *Working Woman*, May, 29–30.

Badger, J. 1995. "Tips for Managing Stress on the Job." *American Journal of Nursing*, September, 31–33.

Beakley, P. 1998. "Are You Smart Enough for Your Job?" *University of Phoenix* (spring): 14–16.

Bernard, L., and Walsh, M. 1996. *Leadership: The Key to Professionalization of Nursing*. New York: Mosby.

Beyers, M. 1996. "The Value of Nursing." *Hospitals and Health Networks*, 5 February, 52.

Bolen, D., and Unland, J. 1994. "Surviving Stress." *Hospitals and Health Networks*, 20 October, 100.

Bridges, W. 1980. *Transitions*. Boston: Addison Wesley Publishing.

———. 1988. *Surviving Corporate Transition*. New York: Doubleday.

Brock, R. 1996. "Head for Business." *Hospitals and Health Networks*, 5 December, 62–66.

California Nurses Association. Web Site Home Page. http://www.califnurses.org/

Collins, H.L. 1989. "How Well Do Nurses Nurture Themselves?" *RN*, May, 39–41.

Conti, R. 1996. "Nurse Case Manager Roles: Implications for Practice." *Nursing Administration Quarterly* 21:1.

Davis, C., ed. 1996. *Nursing Staff in Hospitals and Nursing Homes: Is It Adequate?* National Institute of Medicine. Washington, D.C.: National Academy Press.

Dracup, K., and Bryan-Brown, C., eds. 1998. "Thinking Outside the Box and Other Resolutions." *American Journal of Critical-Care*, January, 1.

Federwisch, A. 1997. "Teammates or Adversaries? Your Attitude Matters." *NurseWeek*, 13 October, 1.

———. 1998. "Attitude Matters." *NurseWeek*, 26 January, 13.

Flower, J. 1997. "Job Shift." *Healthcare Forum Journal*, January/February, 15–24.

Fralicx, R., and Bolster, C.J. 1997. "Preventing Culture Shock." *Modern Healthcare*, 11 August, 50.

Gray, B.B. 1994. "Twenty-First Century Hospital Embodies New Concept." *NurseWeek*, 1 April, 1.

———. 1998. "Are Nurses Credible?" *NurseWeek*, 23 March, 4.

Groves, M. 1996. "Life After Layoffs." *Los Angeles Times*, 25 March, 3.

Hagland, M. 1995. "Incent Me." *Hospitals and Health Networks*, 5 September, 7.

Hammers, M.A. 1994. "Crystal Ball Gazing with Leland Kaiser." *RN Times*, 5 September, 8–10.

Izzo, J. 1998. "The Changing Values of Workers." *Healthcare Forum Journal*, May/June, 62–65.

Jaffe, D., and Scott, C. 1997. "The Human Side of Reengineering." *Healthcare Forum Journal*, September/October, 14–21.

Kanter, R.M. 1983. *The Change Masters*. New York: Simon and Schuster.

Kennedy, M.M. 1996. "Skills Transfer." *Executive Female*, September/October, 27–31.

Kunen, J. 1996. "The New Hands-Off Nursing." *Time*, 30 September, 55–57.

Linden, A. 1998. "Getting What You Want," *Executive Female*, February, 1998, 4–7.

Maltais, M. 1998. "Leadership's Leading Indicators." *Los Angeles Times*, 8 June, 3.

Manion, J. 1996. "Understanding the Seven Stages of Change." *RN Magazine*, April, 21.

Marks, M. 1994. *From Turmoil to Triumph*, New York, Lexington Press.

McLaughlin, P., and McLaughlin, P., Jr. 1998. "The Seven Steps to Top Performance." *Executive Female*, April, 6–8.

Meissner, J. 1986. "Nurses: Are We Eating Our Young?" *Nursing 86,* March, 52–53.

National Association of Female Executives. 1990. *How to Short-Circuit Stress*. Pamphlet. New York: NAFE.

———. 1993. *Guide to a Winning Resume*. Pamphlet. New York: NAFE.

Neale, M. 1997. "The Art of the Deal." *Hospitals and Health Networks*, 5 April, 38–39.

Organization of Nurse Leaders. 1995. "Focus Group Notes." *Nursing Issues*, 29 September.

Perryman, A. 1998. "Sixteen Ways To Succeed in a New Work Place." *Executive Female*, 14 April, 4–7.

Pew Health Professions Commission. 1995. "Healthy America: Practitioners for 2005." *Pew Health Professions Report*. Washington, D.C.: Pew Health Professions Commission.

———. 1998. *"Pew Health Professions Report*. Washington, D.C.: Pew Health Professions Commission.

Public Policy Institute of California. 1996. *Nursing Staff Trends in California Hospitals: 1977–1995*. October. Sacramento, California: Public Policy Institute of California.

Ryan, R. 1998a. "Moving into Management." *Executive Female*, February, 8.

———. 1998b. "Super Effective Interview Tactics." *Executive Female*, February, 6.

Sampson, E. 1996. "Disease State Management: New Models for Case Management." *The Remington Report*, September/October, 21–25.

Sherer, J. 1994a. "Job Shifts." *Hospitals and Health Networks*, 5 October, 64–68.

———. 1994b. "Union Uprising: California Nurses React Aggressively to Work Redesign." *Hospitals and Health Networks*, 20 December, 36–38.

Shindul-Rothschild, J. et al. 1997. "Ten Keys to Quality Care." *American Journal of Nursing* 97(11): 35–43.

Smith, L. 1993. "Never Fail To Be Gracious." *Executive Female*, September/October, 7–10.

Sokolosky, V. 1996. "Mastering Career Change." *Spirit* (Southwest Airlines), August, 132–133.

Stern, C. 1994. "Communication Strategies." Lecture handouts, September 1996, Los Angeles.

Stern, C. et al. 1991. *Kaiser Foundation Hospitals Graduate Nurse Handbook of Job Searching Techniques.* 4th ed. Oakland, California: Kaiser Permanente Hospitals.

Thomas, D. 1994. "Five Ways to Run Your Career Like a Business." *Executive Female,* November/December, 37–40.

Turner, S.O. 1995a. "Marketing Yourself in the 'Nineties." *American Journal of Nursing,* January, 20–23.

———. 1995b. "Stand Out or Lose Out." *Nursing 95*, January, 13–18.

———. 1995c. "Laid Off: Now What?" *Nursing 95*, May, 94–95.

———. 1995d. "Reality Check: It's Time for Nursing to Face the Future." *Hospitals and Health Networks*, 20 August, 20–22.

Van, S. 1994. "A New Attitude." *RN Times*, November, 12–13.

Vitale, S. 1995. "Reinventing Your Career." *Executive Female*, September–October, 43–56.

Woodward, H. 1994. *Navigating Through Change.* Berkeley, California: Richard D. Irwin, Inc.

## CHAPTER 15

# Practical Advice on Career Development: Strategies for a Managed Care Environment

> Become the best you can be in your present role. Exemplify an indispensable employee. These ideas may sound a little corny, but they are important precursors to successful career planning and management.

**CAREER DEVELOPMENT**

Career development means making the decision to take total responsibility for your career and your life! Career success does not just happen—it requires careful planning and analysis. Career development is not necessarily structured as a ladder with different roles at higher and higher levels. Actually, it may be more like a tree, where different branches mean different options and choices, all of them valuable.

Nurses must become active in their own career development. Before you begin, take stock of where you are in your present job. Are you doing your best? Are you enthusiastic? Start the career planning process by identifying your personal and professional goals. There are many variations of the career planning process, but the one I like best is from the *Foundation Hospitals Graduate Nurse Handbook of Job Searching Techniques* (Stern et al, 1991). Use this career planning process to begin managing your career.

First, assess where you are. Determine what you like about your present role and what you don't like. Think about the kinds of things that make you happy in your work. Be honest with yourself. Next, explore what you want and like in a job. Consider all issues and be open-minded and nontraditional in your assessments. (See Exhibit 15–1.)

Gather information about the roles you like. Look at nursing journals and advertisements; talk to colleagues at work and at conferences about what their jobs include. After gathering information on many job options, you can target one or two roles to aim for. The roles you choose should excite you professionally and fit in well with your personal life choices. I have learned the hard way that it is advisable to fit your job around your life instead of your life around your job!

Your next step is to decide on one role to actually pursue. Get as much detailed information as you can, including job requirements, training, potential positions, and salary ranges. You may want to set up an informational interview with one or two nurses who are presently in the role you are interested in.

You then need to develop personal strategies to meet the goal of achieving that role or job. Consider whether you need to go back to school, pick up some continuing education courses, or change your schedule to accomplish the strategies. Include back-up plans and use a flexible approach when developing those strategies. Talk with your nurse manager about your plans. Get your manager's advice and support before you begin.

You are then ready to implement your strategies. Actually implementing your strategies is different than simply planning them. This is the time you put your energy and resources where your mouth is! Make sure your mentors and supervisors know you are actively pursuing career development plans—most of the time they will support and assist you in achieving your goal.

Continue your ongoing career management. Acknowledge yourself and your needs. Write a personal mission statement. Acknowledge what you are not and what you cannot do. This is as important as being aware of your strengths. Identify the role you would have in three years if you could have anything you wanted. Write long-range goal statements with deadlines (for example, "By 200X, I will be _____"). Set short-term goals for one year (for example, "By _____, I will have _____").

Reprogram yourself to attain the goals you have set. Role model your goals to yourself. Remember to reward yourself for successes. Assess your career annually on your birthday and consult with your mentors periodically, or at least yearly. Career planning is an active function you should never delegate or delay!

**Exhibit 15–1**  Self-Assessment Tool

---

1. The tasks/components I like most about my present job are: _____
_____
_____
_____

2. The tasks/components I like least about my present job are: _____
_____
_____
_____

3. My educational goals are: _____
_____
_____

4. My short-term (within one year) goal(s) is (are): By _____, 200__ I will
have: _____
_____
_____

5. My long-term (two–three years) goal(s) is (are): By _____, 200__ I will
have: _____
_____
_____

6. Jobs outside acute care that interest me are: _____
_____
_____

7. Areas of cross-training within the hospital that interest me are: _____
_____
_____

8. The steps I need to take to achieve my short-term goal(s) are: _____
_____
_____

9. The resources I need to achieve my short-term goal(s) are: _____
_____
_____

*Source:* Copyright © 1994, Turner Healthcare Associates, Inc.

## EFFECTIVE INTERVIEWING

If you understand the underlying agenda of the interview process, you will always know how to best articulate your response. It will be difficult for anyone to throw you off with a difficult question. The many questions in an interview all really boil down to only two points: Will you fit in well with this organization? Does this organization suit your skills, interests, personality traits, and values?

If you can answer these two questions, you will give the employer an indication of how well you will perform in that organization. In order to prepare for the interview, you must have a thorough knowledge of the employer and of yourself. The more you know about yourself and why you want to work at this job for this employer, the easier the interview will be.

To prepare adequately for an interview, there are certain types of information you need to learn about the company prior to your meeting. Ideally, you should know the answers to the following questions:

1. Which employers hire people in this industry?
2. How can I make contacts in this industry?
3. Of the employers that hire in this industry, which will I match well with in terms of my skills, values, interests, and personality traits?
4. Will I be happy and effective working for this particular employer?
5. Are there openings in this organization? How do I find out?
6. How does this employer treat employees?
7. What are the opportunities for advancement? For women?
8. How well is this employer/organization doing financially?
9. How does this organization rank within the industry?
10. Does this organization have problems that my skills can help to solve?
11. What are all the services offered by this organization?
12. What is the general image of the organization in the public's mind?
13. What kind of turnover of staff has this organization had?
14. What is the attitude of employees toward the organization?
15. Is promotion generally from within, or from the outside?
16. Does the organization encourage its employees to further their education? Help pay for it?
17. How does the organization communicate within the internal structure? externally?

18. How essential is my position to the organization?
19. What is the reputation of the top management team?
20. What type of management style does the management team have? My potential boss?

You can find much of this information in annual reports, directories, books, newspapers, magazines, newsletters, lists of employers by industry, and professional association directories.

The list of possible questions an applicant is asked in an interview is endless, but they often come down to asking the same thing in several different ways. Remember that questions about your past are really about your future. Try to understand the real intent of a question. When asked about past experience, emphasize skills and achievements. Give specific examples of what you did. The following are a few of the most typically asked questions and suggested responses.

1. "Tell me about yourself."

Talk about your job-related skills. In your mind, consider the question in relation to the job for which you are applying. Do not ask for clarification. This is a typical opener question through which the interviewer gains insight into you. Personal, job-related, or academic experiences are fine to discuss as long as they relate directly to how you will perform the job.

2. "Why do you want this job?"

Be honest, and draw upon the research you have done on the employer as well as on your own self-assessment of skills and experiences as they relate to the position you are interviewing for.

3. "What do you know about this position or employer?"

It is crucial here to have done your homework prior to the interview. You must know about the employer, and it is even more important to know about the position itself. You must have researched the employer and the position prior to the interview to adequately prepare an answer for this question.

4. "What are your strengths?"

Be sure to identify your strengths by using specific skill statements. You will need to complete your own skill self-assessment prior to the interview.

5. "What are your weaknesses?"

Here you are trying to get across the fact that any weakness you have will not affect your ability to do the job. Either identify a weakness that does not directly relate to the work or identify a weakness that you have and explain how you are working on it. Sometimes, you can make a statement about a weakness that actually sounds like a strength. For example, you might respond with a statement that you become frustrated with people who don't think as rapidly as you do.

6. "Where do you see yourself in two years? five? 10?"

Rely on the research you have done about the organization to describe how you plan to develop your skills within the typical career ladder of this organization. Avoid identifying goals that will not benefit the employer.

7. "We have other equally qualified candidates. Why should we select you over the others?"

Again, the most powerful information you can offer is a reiteration of your best skills to perform the job. Realize that your enthusiasm and desire for the position are also convincing.

8. "Do you have any questions?"

Prepare questions ahead of time. Asking intelligent questions reflects the depth of your research and the clarity of your thinking. When you say: "No, my questions have all been answered," you forfeit an opportunity to sell yourself to the employer through the caliber of the questions you ask.

9. "What salary are you looking for?"

Do not inquire about salary during the initial interview; realize, however, that the employer may bring up the subject. Delay salary negotiation until the employer is convinced the organization must have you. Ask to discuss salary when you are both certain you are right for the job. If pressed for an amount, you are best off discussing a salary range, which you will know from your pre-interview research.

To best prepare yourself for the interview, assess your skills, interests, values, and personality traits. Review typical questions and answers to interview questions, as discussed above. Also consider questions you want to ask of the employer. For example:

- To whom would I report?
- Will I get the opportunity to meet that person?
- Where is the job located?
- What are the travel requirements, if any?
- How regularly do performance evaluations occur?
- What nursing or organizational model does your facility follow?
- In researching the position, I discovered that your department has been working on a _____ project. Can you tell me more about this?

Your mother was right: first impressions matter and they are very important. They include non-verbal communications such as body language, eye contact, and voice quality. Sit erect and settled against the back of the chair with an alert, interested expression. Keep your arms relaxed and your hands resting quietly on the chair or in your lap. Cross your legs only at the ankles. Keep your feet on the floor.

Dress to reflect how you want to be perceived, as a professional. Select an understated outfit and accessories that convey your competency. Wear conservative clothing that is appropriate for the interview and your weight. Buy one good navy blue or black suit for all interviews. Buy a full-length mirror and check it before you leave your house. Check front and back views for a tasteful, appropriate appearance.

Smile. Emphasize your confidence and professionalism by smiling often, but appropriately. Use a firm handshake. Grip the interviewer's hand firmly, look into his or her eyes, and say his or her name when introduced and leaving the interview. Maintain eye contact. Always focus on the interviewer in order to draw attention to what you are saying.

Show respect. Let employers make their own judgments—do not share negative comments about old bosses or companies. Avoid using "puff" statements, such as "They couldn't have kept the company without me" or "You'll never get anyone as good as me," when you are closing the interview. Know which questions you must answer and which are illegal (age, marital status, children, race, religion, sexual preference, or personal habits). Be prepared to address concerns about child care by responding that you have reliable child care coverage; there's no need to be defensive.

It may be helpful to review a book on job interviewing. There are many to choose from. To maximize your time at the interview, do some advance preparation before your meeting. As soon as possible, analyze the job and company. Call any contact you have to get an insider perspective. Use the Internet to download information. Learn what the company does and know its products or services. Local libraries often have newspaper archives where you can look up articles on recent developments within the company or in the specific industry.

Get a job description. Call the human resources department and ask them to fax you a complete up-to-date job profile. Learn as much as you can about the job requirements. Ask specific questions about the position, including who you will report to, what the expectations are, and what the greatest challenges are.

It may be useful to create an agenda for yourself. List the top five selling points about you for the job. For example, if you were interviewing for a case management position, you would want to include any previous patient education experience. Compose a short 60-second statement about your strengths and practice it several times. This is a perfect response to questions such as "Tell me about yourself," "What are your strengths?" or "Why should I hire you?" It is also the best way to summarize at the end of an interview.

Gather evidence of your talents and skills. Be ready to show visual examples of your work. Displaying a spreadsheet or project business plan is much more influential than just talking about it. Practice succinct answers to potentially tough questions such as "Why do you want to leave your job?" or "What are your weaknesses?" Effective responses are much easier to compose when you are not on the hot seat to provide them. Practice your delivery with a friend by role playing, or use a video camera or tape recorder to hear how you sound.

Offer only solid references. Notify references beforehand and ask permission to use their names. Prepare a list of those who have either supervised you or dealt with you extensively and can give a firsthand report on your job performance. Offer examples of past successes. Employers hire based on their estimation that what you have done in the past indicates how you will perform for them.

During the interview, your responses to questions should take 60 seconds or less. One-word answers are too short, but lengthy, wandering replies will lose the interviewer's interest. Listen carefully and answer questions directly. If you are unclear on anything, ask for clarification before you give your answer. Create conversations and build rapport by asking a few questions as you go. If you have discussed specific skills, such as patient education or computer literacy, inquire about the systems they use. Then respond with related experience and skills you have to offer.

Demonstrate interest and enthusiasm. A monotone or poker face will not convince the interviewer you are a strong contender. Radiate interest, energy, and confidence. Offer past performance examples to show how you will succeed in this role. Before you leave, tell the interviewer you are very interested in the position.

Thank the interviewer for meeting with you. Before you leave , ask what the next step will be and when you can expect to know the result of the interview. If you don't hear by the stated time frame, call back. It shows interest in the job.

Always, no matter what, type or write a thank-you note to the interviewer within 48 hours of your interview. Take their business card so you will have the proper title and correct spelling and address. Define three or four points that demonstrate why you would succeed at this job. In addition, make four points clear in your letter:

1. You paid attention to what was being said.
2. You understood the importance of the interviewer's comments.
3. You are excited about the job, can do it, and want it.
4. You have good communication skills.

Also, if necessary, correct any negative impressions or clear up confusing issues that surfaced during the interview.

Use key words and phrases in your letter. Words like "recognize," "listen," "enthusiastic," "impressed," "challenge," "confidence," "interest," and "appreciation" can convey your abilities to do the job. Always thank the interviewer for the opportunity, even if it is a job you no longer want. That courtesy may be remembered for a better job in the future.

## CREATING AND USING YOUR RESUME

A resume represents you as a potential job candidate and a professional. It serves several purposes, including application for a job, consideration

---

Interview Checklist

- Make the interview appointment.
- Wear an appropriate suit.
- Prepare an up-to-date resume.
- Learn background information on the facility.
- Ask specific job description and accountability questions.
- Take the interviewer's business card.
- Write a thank-you note to the interviewer.
- Make a follow-up phone call.

for an interview, and creating a first impression when you cannot meet face to face.

Keep your resume brief, neat, and grammatically correct. One typewritten page is preferable; two is maximum. Keep it updated and always have a few on hand ready to send out if needed. Make sure your career objective, if you state one, speaks to the contribution you will make to the organization rather than to how your personal career goals will be met. Use action words such as "developed," "managed," and "created" to highlight your problem-solving abilities, rather than simply recite a litany of job duties. Emphasize accomplishments whenever possible by tying your job responsibilities to quantifiable results achieved.

Include a cover letter, even with a faxed resume. Always. An effective cover letter is a sales letter. It is a second chance, apart from your resume, to sell yourself to an employer. If the letter is effective, it will convince the employer to turn the page to read your resume. A cover letter is also a letter of introduction. It introduces you and your background to the employer.

The letter must have a professional, business-letter format. Each copy must be an original, and use the same paper and type of font as with your resume. Never address a cover letter to "To whom it may concern," "Sir," or "Madam." It will be ineffective to send the same cover letter with just the addressee names changed to a variety of employers. Employers can spot a generic letter a mile away. In addition, don't duplicate the information on your resume in your cover letter. Instead, use the letter as an opportunity to sell your background and experience as it relates to the specific job opening and the hiring organization.

Consider overhauling a "tired" resume if after several months you have received little or no response. It is commonly believed that an effective resume should elicit a 1 percent response. Don't forget that the resume is only the appetizer—say just enough about your qualifications and experience to whet the interviewer's appetite. Once an employer wants to know more about you, you have earned the interview you intended to get.

Do not list salary history or requirements even when asked for. This puts you at an unfair advantage and allows the hiring company to rule you out based on salary alone. But don't ignore the request, either. Instead, make a statement in your cover letter, such as, "Salary requirements will be provided if a mutual interest exists." Try not to discuss salary in an interview until after a job offer has been made.

Don't enclose your list of references with your resume. Have them typed and ready to hand the interviewer if he or she requests them at the meeting. Always call prospective references before listing them to ask permission. Also, don't put too much information on any one page of your resume. Leave some "white" space on the page. Follow up any faxed resume with an original version. This will ensure its receipt and gives you another opportunity to get your resume noticed.

Contents of a resume include a heading, education, experience, and licensure. Resumes can also include professional activities, awards and honors, or languages spoken. The heading should include your name, street address, city, state, and zip code. No abbreviations are appropriate other than those for states. A current telephone number, including area code, is mandatory. Do not write the word "telephone." It is important that employers be able to reach you, or leave a message for you, at the number you have indicated. If you have an answering machine, record a message appropriate for a prospective employer to hear. A serious, business-like message is best.

The education section should include college degrees and dates awarded or expected, institutions from which degrees were/will be attained, and the city and state of each institution. The experience section should include previous positions held. For each position, include job title, name of employer, city and state of employer. Describe the skills used on the job. Start each description with a past tense action verb. Include scope and numbers wherever possible. Avoid beginning descriptions with phrases such as "responsible for,", assisted," and "duties included."

The activities and awards sections can be combined. Include organizations' names, offices held (if any), and dates of membership under the activities. Awards and honors should include the award title, distinction recognized by the award, and the bestowing organization.

There are several resume formats to choose from. The chronological format has experience organized by date, most recent first, and by position. This is the most common resume layout. Use a chronological format if you are entering the job market after many years or for the first time, or are changing fields. In the functional format, experience is organized by function or task. Positions, places of employment, and dates are listed together toward the end of the resume. This design is most appropriate when you do not have specific experience for a particular job, but do have experience that may be relevant. This may be the best format for individuals desiring a career change.

Try to personalize your resume. Not all resumes contain the same categories. Establish categories that best fit your work background and your objective. For example, "experience" may also be titled "employment," "professional experience," etc. Place the categories in the order most relevant to your objective. Page layout includes methods of highlighting important information by means of various type fonts, underlining, bolding, capitalizing, and use of blank space. Use clear, easy-to-read, traditional styles of type font. Use a laser printer or have your resume typeset. Choose high-quality heavy bond paper. Use white, ivory, or light gray color paper. Use a 9 ×12 envelope rather than a traditional business envelope to avoid folding your resume and cover letter. Make sure there are no typographical or spelling errors in your resume or cover letter. These give employers a reason to reject your application. Proof your work carefully!

## ENTERING THE WORK FORCE AFTER TAKING TIME OFF

Many nurses take several years off to have children, and want to return to the work force when their children are older. After a few years staying at home, you may feel awkward and unclear as to how to begin the process of going back to work. While you may have been very accomplished in your last job, your confidence in your abilities may now be a bit shaky and you may not be informed as to what is going on in the industry. You may think potential employers won't give you a chance.

Relax! You can get prepared and psych yourself up at the same time. A big part of returning to the workplace is convincing yourself that you still have what it takes. Don't become your own worst enemy by second-guessing yourself. Keep in mind that if you look, sound, and act confident about your abilities, employers will likely believe in you.

To gain a quick boost of confidence, try to refresh your knowledge of the health care industry. Spend some time at a health care library or on the Internet reading back issues of health care journals and doing basic industry research. Reconnect with former coworkers if you haven't kept in contact and ask them to update you on health care happenings and company gossip. Tell them you are considering going back to work and ask them to keep their ears open for opportunities that may suit you.

No matter what your nursing specialty is, you will need some basic computer skills. It is advisable to enroll in a computer course. Nursing journals often have advertisements for these types of classes. It also impresses potential employers that you are willing to bring your skills up to speed. When you enroll in the course, don't forget to take advantage of schmooze time before and after the class to make new contacts who may know of job opportunities.

You need to overcome the time-off handicap. This fear is not completely unwarranted; it may indeed be tough to get some employers to see beyond the gap in your work history. However, specialty nursing skills are always in demand, and most employers know that nursing shortages are cyclic. You need to make a strong positive impression on potential employers before they ever see your resume. This means networking and making personal connections first.

You can contact potential employers by going to nursing career fairs or specialty conferences. Employers too busy to take your calls in their office will now be colleagues you can talk with during breaks in the conferences. Ask them if they have openings or know of other job options available. Bring business cards with your name, address, and telephone number on them, and don't forget to send follow-up notes and thank them for their time and assistance.

Informational interviews are another way to introduce yourself to potential employers. Call health care facilities where you would like to work and schedule an informational meeting with the supervisor of the area you are interested in. Ask her how she got her position and what qualifications are required to work there. Tell her a little bit about your background and ask what you could do to work in that area. You don't want to ask directly for a job during these meetings, but chances are, if you have made a good impression, the manager will tell you about any current or anticipated job openings.

You may also network via the Web. Many health care facilities have Web sites that post job opportunities, as well as the names of key employees. Don't be shy about writing to some of these people and having an e-mail discussion about the company, job opportunities, and your areas of nursing expertise.

Last but not least, revamp your resume. When it is time to send in your resume, reorganize it so that it is skill-based rather than chronological. The best facilities to approach if you are reentering the work force may be small companies with flexible hiring policies, women-owned or women-directed businesses, and facilities with a reputation for family-friendliness.

## SUCCESS STRATEGIES FOR YOUR NEW ROLE

There are strategies you can use to be successful in a new workplace. If you can implement these strategies, chances are you will be very successful in your new role. One good thing about starting a new job or moving to a new work site is the opportunity it gives you to become the person and the employee you really want to be perceived as. A career change allows you the chance to review the skills and attitudes that have worked both for and against you in the past. It also gives you a chance to demonstrate the best of what you have learned and observed from your past experience.

Try to consider the change that is taking place an opportunity for both personal and professional growth. Your work site is a collection of experiences and learning resources. You can challenge yourself to learn and use as many of these as possible.

Come up with ideas of how to do your job better and more efficiently. Try not to get tied into a particular set of tasks and skills too closely. Be aware that the current rate of change may limit you if your focus is too narrow.

Watch stereotypes and don't believe everything you hear. People can go from clinical areas to management and be good managers. Leadership skills are not based on gender or cultural background. Having children is not necessarily a prerequisite for understanding the needs and circumstances of working parents. Make your own decision about the strengths and weaknesses of your new manager or nursing colleagues.

Be careful how you speak. Present positive messages that are articulate, succinct, and appropriate. Good manners still matter. Work on listening skills. This requires basic receptiveness to new ideas and concepts that may not match your perceptions.

Learn as much as you can on your own. Practice figuring out how to achieve something instead of thinking up reasons it can't be done. Try to use past experience to benefit you in your new role without being focused on the "way you have always done it."

Ask for feedback from supervisors, managers, and nursing peers. Take an active role in creating a positive image of who you are and what you can accomplish. Find a mentor and work with that person to network and achieve your career goals.

## WHEN YOUR CAREER IS SIDELINED

Nothing strikes terror in an employee's heart as quickly as finding herself increasingly out of the loop. You have seen the signs; you may even have been affected by them. The sidelining process works like this: An employee is treated as if she were an automaton with no opinions or feelings about anything that matters at work. People move around her as if she was an obstacle in the road. She is informed of important decisions only after the fact. It is as if the employee played no active role in the life of the organization. Without ongoing contact with other workers, performance will decline as more and more of the information along the grapevine skips her.

According to Marilyn Moats Kennedy (Kennedy, 1996b), employees can be sidelined and pushed out of the mainstream without being aware it is happening. The organization will only tolerate an employee out of the mainstream for a short period of time before the employee is terminated or laid off. Consider some of these questions posed by Kennedy:

1. Has anything happened on the job in the past week that surprised you?
2. Do people stop talking when you approach?
3. Are your decisions overruled by your peers?
4. Does your boss send you messages through your subordinates?
5. Are you rarely asked for your opinion or input?
6. Are your telephone calls returned less and less promptly?
7. Do people request voice mail rather than try to reach you directly? (Kennedy, 1996b)

If you answered yes to some of these questions, your job may be at risk! If you have "pulled back" at work, it may be evident to those around you. Workers choose to withdraw for different reasons. It may be because the worker is considering a job change, has personal problems, or has given up on the organization. The trouble is that realizing one is on the outside comes so gradually it may be imperceptible until an event makes it plain to all. Then, it is usually too late. Hanging back, withdrawing from the fray, or just hiding out in your work space should be warning signs that you are courting burnout or your problems are beginning to show, according to Kennedy.

You need to take action. Talk to your boss, and buy some time. Reestablish contact with coworkers. Most importantly, don't kid yourself about the seriousness of what is happening to you. The longer the inaction, the fewer the choices. At least 10 percent of people who have been downsized were laid off because they had withdrawn, not because their jobs were eliminated (Kennedy, 1996a).

If you are downsized or laid off, you need to be prepared to deal with that, too. Consider the items on this checklist to protect yourself after a layoff.

- Don't panic.
- Remember, it isn't disciplinary.
- Don't get angry with your supervisor or the person who tells you.
- Don't discuss severance at first meeting. If possible, reschedule when you are not in shock.
- Create a resume and keep it up-to-date.
- Document as much as you can about your layoff meeting. It is all right to take notes.
- Meet with Human Resources to review current benefit status.
- Ask for outplacement service, especially in lieu of severance (outplacement provides help finding another job, and resources to use during the process, such as phones, offices, and resume assistance).
- Negotiate hard for severance. Usual rule of thumb is one week per year of service.
- Apply quickly for unemployment; it takes time to get payments through the bureaucracy.
- Leave the same day and take all your belongings. It's too painful to come back later.
- Don't take hospital property or erase computer files. These can be prosecuted as criminal offenses, and at the very least will harm your chances of good references later.
- Ask for written references from Human Resources and your supervisor.
- Keep an updated list of professional references.
- Tell everyone you are looking for a job.
- Keep in contact with colleagues.

- Take special care of yourself and try to use what you have the most of: TIME!
- Review books and articles on resume writing, interviewing, career choices.
- Do not burn your bridges by publicly complaining about your previous employer.
- Remember, you are not what you do! ( See "Coping with Downsizing" in Chapter 14.)

## MASTERING CAREER CHANGE

According to experts, the average person experiences six to eight job changes in a lifetime, either as a matter of choice or involuntarily. In the early 1990s, about 12 million people were switching to new careers. By the year 2000, fifty million people will be challenging the tradition of a once-in-a-lifetime career. Half of those leave jobs involuntarily (see, you are not the only one!), either because the job is being phased out or because of a performance problem. The others have moved on because the job is a wrong fit or the individual is disillusioned with the company.

To survive and thrive in a job change, we need to develop and refine our problem-solving skills and levels of thinking. An attitude of constant willingness to learn makes you more employable. Keep self-confidence up by realizing you are selling something—yourself. Think of yourself as a valuable resource rather than someone begging for an opportunity. While coaches and counselors can share their ideas for direction, no one can walk in your shoes but you. Look at your resume as well as your current competencies and skills. Decide for yourself what actions and goals to achieve. Qualities during career change include personal energy and drive, self-confidence, commitment to a long-term involvement, problem-solving ability, understanding of how to use resources, and ability to use positive and negative feedback wisely.

## TREAT YOUR CAREER LIKE A BUSINESS BY MANAGING IT

According to Dan Thomas in an *Executive Female* article (November/ December 1994), many people do not use good business sense in managing their careers. Over the years he has observed that the best students and best managers are not always the most successful in their own careers.

Why? What is it that makes the most difference between success and failure in a career? Is it contacts, luck, or just hard work? Any or all of those can help, but no single specific factor is the determining factor.

Thomas believes there are specific things you can do to improve the chances of success in your career. The first two are particularly crucial, especially since few people give them any thought. First, choose the right business. Many people don't recognize what seems an obvious conclusion: whenever you have the choice, it's always better to choose a great business or organization. What's the difference? Great businesses have three characteristics: growth potential, profit potential, and diversification potential. Growth potential is the most important characteristic according to Thomas.

Second, create the right strategy. Strategy consists of the decisions you make to position yourself in a complex environment (which certainly characterizes health care). You can choose to manage this strategy actively or to abdicate responsibility and let your environment make decisions for you. Many people erroneously think that if they do a good job, they will be successful. You need to market yourself by differentiating your skills so that what you have to offer is uniquely important to the organization you work in.

Third, develop the right systems. There is no such thing as job security. Information is a crucial component of what you need to be successful. Having the right information at the right time is very important. Many people measure their career success on past performance, which is only part of the picture. As important as it is to look backward, it is more important to look ahead to see what is coming down the road. Identify the skills and abilities of the people at your level in your industry. What are leaders in your organization and industry doing to develop themselves and stay ahead of the competition? Read as much as you can and talk to those who know to find out what skills nurses of the future will need. Then you will know how to market yourself.

Fourth, design the right support structure. Individuals need a support structure of mentors, colleagues, and subordinates to help them achieve their objectives. Mentors can be active or passive. Active mentors are those who are willing to coach you as you progress. Passive mentors are role models you can emulate. You most likely need both in nursing. Colleagues and subordinates who can cooperate with you and have complementary skills can be sources for future success (Thomas, 1994).

## COMMUNICATION SKILLS FOR NURSES

There are numerous and complex definitions for communication. It is a vital process, not a static one. It is constantly changing. Communication is usually defined as the sending and receiving of information, feelings, and attitudes, both verbally and non-verbally, that produces a response (Bernard and Walsh, 1996).

In effective communication, a message is transmitted and received, but real communication occurs once the receiver provides some response to the sender. Here is a specific communication sequence of events. There are many different models to explain the communication sequence; however, all models provide these essential elements or components.

Elements of Communication:
• sender or encoder
• receiver
• message (the meaning the sender wants to send)
• symbols (how message is sent—e.g., verbal, non-verbal)
• message (the meaning actually received)

Communication Sequence:
Sender⟹ Meaning⟹ Message⟹ Symbols⟹ Meaning⟹ Receiver

Effective communication exists between two persons when the receiver interprets the sender's message in the same way the sender intended it. The sender is affected by his or her personal background, attitudes, perceptions, emotions, opinions, education, and experience. There is a specific meaning in the message that the sender intends to send. There are symbols used to communicate, both verbal and non-verbal. The message has meaning when the message is actually received by the recipient. The receiver of the sender's message is also affected by his or her personal background, attitudes, perceptions, emotions, opinions, education, and experience.

It is important to note that the same factors for effective communication can also be barriers to effective communication. For example, a speaker's ethnic background can make that person good at communicating with other members who share the same cultural background; however, this same speaker may not be equally effective when speaking to a culturally diverse audience. Other barriers to effective communication also include:

---

Factors That Affect Communication

- Background (ethnic, cultural)
- Attitudes and values
- Perceptions (conscious impression of the world around us)
- Emotions, level of stress
- Opinions (one's own views and biases)
- Education
- Experience
- Expectations

---

- preconceived assumptions and stereotypes
- distractions (e.g., extraneous noise, other things on your mind, too many people talking at once)
- emotional triggers (e.g., expressing feelings or criticism in statements which create listener resentment, as in "What did you do now?")
- confusing or complex language that has a different meaning to the sender and receiver (such as "Did the patient void?")
- physical barriers (e.g., hearing impairment, poor lighting)
- unpreparedness
- failure to be direct and concise
- feelings of intimidation in a high-pressure environment
- poor timing because the receiver is not ready to listen

Insensitivity can also damage communication by causing the sender or receiver to look at the situation from only one point of view. Non-verbal gestures, movements (tapping, avoiding eye contact), tone, pitch, inflection, and mumbling also cause ineffective communication.

## STRATEGIES TO ENHANCE COMMUNICATION

There are successful strategies nurses can use to enhance communication. During stressful times effective communication becomes critical. Because many nurses are overwhelmed and frustrated by the managed care changes they must deal with, effective communication strategies become even more important. Use an open-ended style of questioning. Open-ended questions are questions requiring more than a yes or no answer. Select the proper environment. Privacy is an important consideration for both nurses and patients as well as anyone involved in a conflict or stressful situation.

Timing is important. It may not be a good idea to bring up a conflict to your boss on a bad day or on her birthday. Be selective when choosing to discuss conflicts. Send your own message by using first-person singular pronouns: "I feel. . . . " This type of personal ownership includes clearly taking responsibility for the ideas and feelings that one expresses. People disown their messages when they use phrases like "most people" or "our group." Such language makes it difficult for listeners to tell whether the individuals really think and feel what they are saying or whether they are repeating thoughts and feelings of others.

Ask for feedback on how your messages are received. To communicate effectively, you must be aware of how the receiver is interpreting and processing your messages. The only way to be sure is to continually seek feedback as to what meanings the receiver is attaching to your messages. Make the message appropriate to the receiver's frame of reference. Use different appropriate words and depths of explanation for an expert in the field and a novice, a child and an adult, your boss and a co-worker.

Non-verbal communication is the most important aspect of communication, and often the most ignored. Body language is 55 percent of communication. Tone of voice is 38 percent. Actual words stated are 7 percent (Bernard and Walsh, 1996). Maintaining good eye contact instills credibility and honesty in the receiver. Make verbal and non-verbal messages consistent and congruent. Every face-to-face communication involves both verbal and non-verbal messages. Usually these messages are congruent. Problems arise when a person's verbal and non-verbal messages are contradictory because the nonverbals do not support the verbals and the receiver is confused.

Make your messages complete and specific. Include clear statements of all necessary information the receiver needs in order to comprehend the message. Being complete and specific seems obvious, but often people do not communicate the frame of reference they are using, the assumptions they are making, the intentions they have in communicating, or the leaps in thinking they are making.

Focus on issues and behaviors, not persons. Describe others' behavior without evaluating or interpreting. When reacting to the behavior of others, be sure to describe their behavior (e.g., *"You keep interrupting me."*) rather than evaluating it (e.g., *"You're a rotten, self-centered egotist who won't listen to anyone else's ideas."*). Get rid of "excess baggage." Learn to minimize redundancy, excessive detail, irrelevant information, and distractions. Outline in your mind what you want to say.

Listening is a critical element of the communication process. Listening skills can be developed. Anyone who wants to get the most out of a dialogue must be both a good speaker and a good listener. Types of listening are defined as passive (listening you don't have to work at, such as to TV and music), and active (where full attention is required in order to hear and understand the whole message).

To be successful at active listening, you must listen for the purpose of understanding what is meant, not for the purpose of readying yourself for a reply. Try to listen to the whole message first; don't interpret too quickly what speaker is trying to say. Attempt to put aside your own views and opinions while actively listening. Put yourself in the speaker's shoes; how does he view the world?

Try to keep your thoughts from being interrupted by how you plan to respond. Don't trust your intuition. Validate the message with the sender. Expect the speaker to use different words than you might and try not to make snap judgments.

An assertive communication style is most effective for making and refusing requests, giving and receiving recognition, and giving and receiving criticism. Assertive communication requires identifying a behavior and defining what is expected. It is often difficult for nurses to communicate assertively without defensiveness. Try using scripting techniques by describing a particular situation or behavior: "When you . . . " Then, express your reactions and feelings: "I feel. . . . " Be specific about the changes you want to occur: "I want you to. . . . "

Nurses often focus on specific behaviors exhibited and not on the entire communication process. Try to identify common goals and outcomes. You could say "If this happens, then. . . . " OR "If you do this, then. . . . "

Aggressive communication is a very strong and powerful communication style. It is usually used with anger. Most people have difficulty dealing with aggressive communication. To handle someone communicating aggressively, try the following steps:

- Dispel any erroneous information.
- Wait until you and they are calm.
- Recognize, feel, and accept your own anger.
- Role play with a safe person.
- Use physical activity to dispel anger.
- Vent anger on an inanimate object.
- In a real situation, express anger in a private, controlled environment.

Nurses can deal with their personal anxiety about anger and aggressive behavior or their own non-assertiveness by:

- relaxation
- avoiding self-defeating thoughts
- desensitization—breaking fear into small bits
- visualization and imagery
- self-coaching and self-talk

## USING POWER TO MANAGE CONFLICT

Power is defined as the ability to control, influence, or act. Authority is defined as the legitimate power granted to an individual by an organization. Power is vested in a position. Leadership is the relationship between two or more people in which one influences the other toward accomplishing a goal without legitimate power.

There are several different types of power, as defined in management textbooks. Personal power is the ability to link the outer capacity for action with the inner capacity of reflection. Organizational power is the ability to accomplish goals through others within an organization. Executive power is the use of personal persuasion and influence to motivate others.

Legitimate power is given to individuals based on their position in an organization. Reward power is the power to provide distribution of rewards. Coercive power is the ability to administer punishment (the opposite of reward). Expert power is earned by an individual with expert knowledge and skills in a certain area or industry. Referent power is the ability to have influence over another based on respect and admiration.

Managers need both power (all types) and authority to be effective. Nurses often see power as bad or negative, but it is a neutral force. People who tend to feel powerless often display the inability to accomplish a goal. Powerless people often resort to other methods to get what they want, such as manipulation, dishonesty, and illegal behaviors. People with power move through stages with that power, beginning with dictatorship, moving to seduction, persuasion, role modeling, and finally to empowerment.

There are several myths about power. These include:

| Myth | Reality |
| --- | --- |
| Power is bad. | Power is neutral. |
| Power is a goal. | Power is a means to accomplish goals. |
| Powerful people are ruthless. | Powerless people are ruthless. |
| Power can be given to others. | Power must be earned or assumed. |
| It is wrong or bad to want power. | Power to accomplish goals can reduce stress and frustration. |

Conflict is inevitable in life and at work due to complex organizations, differing employee interests and needs, and change with transition. Many people are not comfortable with conflict because they have had no training to deal with it. Nurses' schools do not provide training in conflict management or conflict resolution skills.

Conflict may make individuals and groups feel scared and powerless. Conflict is not bad; it is inherently neutral, the same as power. Conflict is not personal, but people often make it personal. Conflict can be functional because it leads to discussion, investigation, and accomplishment of new goals. Excessive conflict can be dysfunctional and lead to strife, not problem solving.

Before resolution can begin, the cause of conflict must be identified. There are different types of conflict. There is conflict within a person or a group, between groups, or between organizations. There are different causes of conflict at work, including goal incompatibility, competition for scarce resources, task interdependencies such as work shared between departments, organizational structure, and integration of roles. Groups are a frequent source of conflict because people come with their own set of values, history, and expectations. Cultural diversity of the nursing work force can also lead to conflict. Communication styles can also cause conflict.

Conflict is over-feared and under-valued! It happens to each of us every day. It is a part of life—from the moment we wake up in the morning, we experience and handle many different types of conflict. Why is it, then, when confronted with conflict in the workplace, most nurses become ineffective? Many nurses would rather avoid conflict altogether than deal with whatever issue causes the tension.

It is unclear to me what makes conflict so difficult for nurses. For some, undoubtedly, fear of the conflict resolution process is the hard part. For others, conflict may always be seen as a negative personal issue, and therefore avoided at all costs. For the profession of nursing, conflict has always been avoided or glossed over and not dealt with. This has caused many formidable and difficult issues to be endlessly debated and never resolved. Consider the sensitive issue of nursing educational preparation. Discussions of this issue have been going on for at least 30 years and there is still no defined, universal entry-into-practice education statement for nursing.

According to Bernard and Walsh (1996) in *Leadership: The Key to the Professionalization of Nursing*, conflict is a normal, unavoidable part of human relationships and can be a growth-producing process if people learn how to manage it effectively. From the perspective of Hitt, Middlemist, and Mathis (1986), although each case of conflict has unique causes, most can be traced to four major sources: goal incompatibility, competition for scarce resources, task interdependencies, and organizational structure.

Conflict exists when two or more parties (individuals, groups, or organizations) differ with regard to facts, opinions, beliefs, feelings, drives, needs, goals, methods, values, or anything else (Bernard and Walsh, 1996). The conflict produced by the differences between these parties creates tension and discomfort. Because of the discomfort conflict causes, most people view conflict as negative, and something to be avoided.

Disagreement between groups about their goals can create conflict, especially if the accomplishment of one group's goals prevents the other group from achieving its goals. Consider a concept like exceptional charting. If you see benefits for you in not implementing exceptional charting, then you will feel conflict if your unit is to transition into exceptional charting practices. Competition for scare resources is an all-too-common theme for conflict in today's health care institutions. Dollars, people, space, and time are all in short supply.

If you depend on another department to help you achieve your goals, conflict will occur if that department achieves a goal that negatively affects your department. For instance, closing the Admitting Office after midnight may be seen as great by the Admitting staff, but as a real inconvenience for the ER night staff.

Most organizational structures also cause conflict to occur. Differing goals, roles, and viewpoints between managers and subordinates, or project managers and operations staff, are common and often difficult to resolve. In this era of health reform and constantly changing environments and circumstances, there is more conflict than ever before!

Gaylyn Mileur, RN, MN, a Director of Nursing for Critical Care and Surgery in New Orleans, believes that nurses are unprepared to handle conflict. "Most nurses are women and women are not brought up to deal with conflict," she says. "Men are socialized to see conflict as a usual occurrence in life, not as a personal attack or unusual situation" (personal communication, 1994). The other big issue that causes nurses to dread dealing with conflict, according to Mileur, is lack of accountability. She states, "Nurses see it easier to avoid conflict because they have no personal accountability for what they believe in. . . . Nurses tend to expect someone else like a labor union or DON to take accountability for nursing issues. . . . The days of the hospital taking care of you forever are over" (personal communication, 1994).

Change causes conflict. It is part of the natural change process. Although individuals can be resistant to the current changes we are seeing in health care, the impetus for change is coming from both outside and inside the industry. Conflict resulting from implementing those changes can resolve differences, clarify issues, and promote unity when managed effectively. To avoid conflict is to eliminate the possibility of defining goals, discussing issues, and designing a unifying philosophy about the issue.

Conflict is about power. If you are a leader who implements change, conflict will inevitably result as a by-product of that change. For a leader to use her power effectively, she must deal with the conflict in order for the change process to take place. To avoid conflict is to ignore the power of leadership. Surrendering power creates ineffective leaders and limits change potential when health care needs it most.

Conflict in and of itself is not bad. It creates tension and makes people feel uncomfortable. Ignoring conflict and tension is what causes poor problem resolution, frustration, and defensiveness. Conflict is often seen as negative. The negativity is not inherent in conflict itself, but rather comes from the tension caused by not handling the original issue.

Vicki Russell, RN, an assistant head nurse in the Critical Care Unit at Valley Presbyterian Hospital in Van Nuys, California, says that "nurses fear conflict because the tension it creates makes them less articulate and the increased stress, workload, and time demands makes any conflict feel personal" (personal communication, 1994).

Conflict enhances advocacy. Above all else, nurses continually strive to be advocates. Patients, families, and the under-served are the recipients of that advocacy. Handling conflict allows advocacy to flourish. To not deal with conflict limits advocacy and intervention effectiveness.

There are two ways to deal with conflict. One way is to utilize conflict resolution. There are different types of conflict resolution techniques, including team building, sharing perspectives non-defensively, attempting to focus on cooperative goals, transition management, education, and communication. Conflict resolution seeks a solution that completely satisfies all parties involved in the conflict. Rarely is it possible to satisfy all the needs of everyone involved. Some compromises are usually made to reach agreement.

The more common way to deal with conflict is through conflict management, which implies a conscious effort to deal with the conflict and control the problem. It does not guarantee to satisfy all involved, but attempts to meet as many needs as possible in determining a solution (Bernard and Walsh, 1996).

There are numerous issues that enter into a conflict situation. The values, goals, resources, and beliefs of the people involved will affect their willingness to compromise and resolve the issues. Past relationships between conflicting parties are also important. If you have no respect for or do not trust your adversary, chances are you will not be committed to managing the conflict.

Nurses apply different strategies to conflict situations. The first choice is often to deny that the conflict exists. This causes no change in the conflict situation at all. If denial doesn't work, some nurses try to ignore conflict. This may relieve tension initially, but the relief is usually short-lived. Ignoring conflict causes relationships to further deteriorate and people will keep feeling bad. Suppressing conflict may be why people think of it as negative and destructive.

While difficult, it is much easier in the long run to deal with conflict head-on. Confrontation means letting the other party know you disagree and being willing to discuss the issues using collaboration, arbitration, problem solving, or compromise. Many nurses who deal with conflict get stuck in the confrontation and never get to the discussion phase.

Not dealing with conflict is the single most limiting factor in resolving nursing issues, at both the local and national levels. The nursing profession has yet to be comfortable with the ideas that conflict is good and creative dissonance is beneficial to addressing changing issues. Instead of dealing with conflict up front, nursing groups tend to "take sides" according to special interests. No formal confrontation takes place, and as a result, the profession is perceived as divisive and splintered in its beliefs and goals.

Physicians seem to be much more comfortable dealing with conflict than nurses. They certainly have just as many issues to disagree on, but physicians are able to "duke it out" behind closed doors and come out with a united stance for their profession. Nurses could learn from that approach. We could be so much more powerful in redesigning health care delivery and health reform systems if the profession was willing to "get down and dirty" to resolve its differences before airing its laundry in public.

The formation of the Federal Nursing Commission for the Institute of Medicine Study is a classic example of not dealing with conflict and going public with the issues before discussion. Chances are no commission would have been needed and almost one million dollars in federal funds could have been saved if nursing representatives could have dealt with the conflicts over staffing, patient care outcomes, and nursing injuries beforehand.

Conflict will always be with us. Nursing will continue to disagree on issues fundamental to the profession and critical to patient advocacy. Resolving conflict takes a strong stomach and the willingness to be uncomfortable. Nurses need to learn to see that differing opinions are not bad, and that dissonance fosters creativity and collaborative outcomes. Nursing has to learn to stop being afraid of conflict and start learning to use it!

## DISCUSSION QUESTIONS

1. Identify appropriate clothing for an interview. Does appearance matter in your geographic area? Why or why not?
2. Are nurses in your geographic area prepared to interview effectively? Why or why not?
3. Role play appropriate and inappropriate interview answers and questions.
4. Do nurses you know have appropriate resumes?

5. List and discuss appropriate resumes. Look at samples. Why are they appropriate?
6. Practice creating an appropriate resume and thank-you note for an interview.
7. Do nurses routinely reenter the work force after taking time off in your geographic area? For what reasons are they likely to take time off?
8. Are they usually successful at reentering the work force? Why or why not?
9. What are the benefits and limitations of hiring and orienting nurses who have been out of the work force for a period of time?
10. Have you ever had your career sidelined? Has anyone you know had theirs sidelined? Why?

---

## BIBLIOGRAPHY

Adizes, S. 1993. *Mastering Change*. Pacific Palisades, California: Adizes Institute Publications.

Austin, N. 1995. "The Skill Every Manager Must Master." *Working Woman*, May, 29–30.

Badger, J. 1995. "Tips for Managing Stress on the Job." *American Journal of Nursing*, September, 31–33.

Beakley, P. 1998. "Are You Smart Enough for Your Job?" *University of Phoenix* (spring): 14–16.

Bernard, L., and Walsh, M. 1996. *Leadership: The Key to Professionalization of Nursing*. New York: Mosby.

Beyers, M. 1996. "The Value of Nursing." *Hospitals and Health Networks*, 5 February, 52.

Bolen, D., and Unland, J. 1994. "Surviving Stress." *Hospitals and Health Networks*, 20 October, 100.

Bridges, W. 1980. *Transitions*. Boston: Addison Wesley Publishing.

————. 1988. *Surviving Corporate Transition*. New York: Doubleday.

Brock, R. 1996. "Head for Business." *Hospitals and Health Networks*, 5 December, 62–66.

California Nurses Association. Web Site Home Page. http://www.califnurses.org/

Collins, H.L. 1989. "How Well Do Nurses Nurture Themselves?" *RN*, May, 39–41.

Conti, R. 1996. "Nurse Case Manager Roles: Implications for Practice." *Nursing Administration Quarterly* 21:1.

Davis, C., ed. 1996. *Nursing Staff in Hospitals and Nursing Homes: Is It Adequate?* National Institute of Medicine. Washington, D.C.: National Academy Press.

Dracup, K., and Bryan-Brown, C., eds. 1998. "Thinking Outside the Box and Other Resolutions." *American Journal of Critical-Care*, January, 1.

Federwisch, A. 1997. "Teammates or Adversaries? Your Attitude Matters." *NurseWeek*, 13 October, 1.

―――. 1998. "Attitude Matters." *NurseWeek,* 26 January, 13.

Flower, J. 1997. "Job Shift." *Healthcare Forum Journal*, January/February, 15–24.

Fralicx, R., and Bolster, C.J. 1997. "Preventing Culture Shock." *Modern Healthcare*, 11 August, 50.

Gray, B.B. 1994. "Twenty-First Century Hospital Embodies New Concept." *NurseWeek*, 1 April, 1.

Groves, M. 1996. "Life After Layoffs." *Los Angeles Times*, 25 March, 3.

Hagland, M. 1995. "Incent Me." *Hospitals and Health Networks*, 5 September, 7.

Hammers, M.A. 1994. "Crystal Ball Gazing with Leland Kaiser." *RN Times*, 5 September, 8–10.

Hitt, M., Middlemist, R., and Mathis, R. 1986. *Management Concepts and Effective Practice*. 2nd ed. Houston, Texas: West Publishing.

Izzo, J. 1998. "The Changing Values of Workers." *Healthcare Forum Journal*, May/June, 62–65.

Jaffe, D., and Scott, C. 1997. "The Human Side of Reengineering." *Healthcare Forum Journal*, September/October, 14–21.

Kanter, R.M. 1983. *The Change Masters*. New York: Simon and Schuster.

Kennedy, M.M. 1996a. "Skills Transfer." *Executive Female*, September/October, 27–31.

―――. 1996b. "When Your Career Is Sidelined." *Executive Female*, September/October, 33–35.

Kunen, J. 1996. "The New Hands-Off Nursing." *Time*, 30 September, 55–57.

Linden, A. 1998. "Getting What You Want." *Executive Female,* February, 1998, 4–7.

Maltais, M. 1998. "Leadership's Leading Indicators." *Los Angeles Times*, 8 June, 3.

Manion, J. "Understanding the Seven Stages of Change." *RN Magazine*, April, 21.

Marks, M. *From Turmoil to Triumph*. 1994. New York: Lexington Press.

McLaughlin, P., and McLaughlin, P., Jr. 1998. "The Seven Steps to Top Performance." *Executive Female*, April, 6–8.

Meissner, J. 1986. "Nurses: Are We Eating Our Young?" *Nursing '86,* March, 52–53.

National Association of Female Executives. 1990. *How to Short-Circuit Stress*. Pamphlet. New York: NAFE.

―――. 1993. *Guide to a Winning Resume*. Pamphlet. New York: NAFE.

Neale, M. 1997. "The Art of the Deal." *Hospitals and Health Networks*, 5 April, 38–39.

Organization of Nurse Leaders. 1995. "Focus Group Notes." *Nursing Issues,* 29 September.

Perryman, A. 1998. "Sixteen Ways To Succeed in a New Work Place. " *Executive Female*, April, 14.

Pew Health Professions Commission. 1995. "Healthy America: Practitioners for 2005." *Pew Health Professions Report*. Washington, D.C.: Pew Health Professions Commission.

————. 1998. *Pew Health Professions Report*. Washington, D.C.: Pew Health Professions Commission.

Public Policy Institute of California. 1996. *Nursing Staff Trends in California Hospitals: 1977–1995*. October. Sacramento, California: Public Policy Institute of California.

Ryan, R. 1998a. "Moving into Management." *Executive Female*, February, 8.

————. 1998b. "Super Effective Interview Tactics." *Executive Female*, February, 6.

Sampson, E. 1996. "Disease State Management: New Models for Case Management." *The Remington Report*, September/October, 21–25.

Sherer, J. 1994a. "Job Shifts." *Hospitals and Health Networks*, 5 October, 64–68.

————. 1994b. "Union Uprising: California Nurses React Aggressively to Work Redesign." *Hospitals and Health Networks*, 20 December, 36–38.

Shindul-Rothschild, J. et al. 1997. "Ten Keys to Quality Care." *American Journal of Nursing* 97(11): 35–43.

Smith, L. 1993. "Never Fail To Be Gracious." *Executive Female*, September/October, 7–10.

Sokolosky, V. 1996. "Mastering Career Change." *Spirit* (Southwest Airlines), August, 132–133.

Stern, C. 1994. "Communication Strategies." Lecture handouts, September 1996, Los Angeles.

Stern, C. et al. 1991. *Kaiser Foundation Hospitals Graduate Nurse Handbook of Job Searching Techniques*. 4th ed. Oakland, California: Kaiser Permanente Hospitals.

Thomas, D. 1994. "Five Ways to Run Your Career Like a Business." *Executive Female*, November/December, 37–40.

Turner, S.O. 1995a. "Marketing Yourself in the 'Nineties." *American Journal of Nursing*, January, 20–23.

————. 1995b. "Stand Out or Lose Out." *Nursing 95*, January, 13–18.

————. 1995c. "Laid Off: Now What?" *Nursing 95*, May, 94–95.

————. 1995d. "Reality Check: It's Time for Nursing to Face the Future." *Hospitals and Health Networks*, 20 August, 20–22.

Van, S. 1994. "A New Attitude." *RN Times*, November, 12–13.

Vitale, S. 1995. "Reinventing Your Career." *Executive Female*, September/October, 43–56.

Woodward, H. 1994. *Navigating Through Change*. Berkeley, California: Richard D. Irwin, Inc.

# CHAPTER 16

# Nurses and Unions: Do They Mix?

Unions have existed in the workplace for over 50 years. Membership has waxed and waned in relation to political environments and the perceived amount of power that unions have over business. In the 1950s, unions were strong and powerful. They became less powerful in the 1970s and 1980s, primarily because of the conservative players in government and alleged Mob connections. In addition, union leaders like William Elder, Chief Operating Officer of the Ventura/Santa Barbara County, California International Brotherhood of Teamsters, acknowledge that the failed air traffic controller strike in the early 1980s damaged union recruiting significantly (personal communication, 1998). Unions have enjoyed a resurgence in the 1990s as industry grapples with economic realities and fewer resources.

Union activity has increased dramatically in the health care field over the past few years. The strategies hospitals created for restructuring have resulted in massive changes for nursing and other hospital employees. Increased health care workplace issues related to staffing mix, staffing ratios, salaries, and benefits have caused nurses to seek assistance from collective bargaining groups. Nurses have turned to different collective bargaining groups for representation. There are groups specifically formed to represent nurses, such as the California Nurses Association or the United Nurses Associations of California. Other collective bargaining groups include nurses in their membership, such as the AFL-CIO and SEIU.

Collective bargaining organizations (unions) exist to create contracts between employers and employees. Unions represent many different types of employees. Each group of employees is called a **bargaining unit**. Contracts are specific to different employee bargaining units. Representatives paid by the union carry on negotiations, represent employees during grievance procedures, and advocate for the work of the organization.

According to Bill Elder, the Secretary/Treasurer for International Brotherhood of Teamsters Local 186, collective bargaining arrangements exist to protect the worker. A collective bargaining arrangement is a contract in which both employers and employees invest their money and time. It clarifies roles, rules, and expectations up front. He believes it eliminates problems and defines what is to be done by both parties. That eliminates confusion, he says, by providing a Bill of Rights for the employee and a explanation of workers' responsibilities for managers.

According to the constitution and bylaws of one collective bargaining organization, the American Federation of Teachers, the objectives of the organization are:

- To promote the organization of all workers in general, and teachers in particular, to impress upon its membership, employers, and the public that it is to the advantage of government, industry, the public, and all concerned that workers be organized.
- To promote the efficiency and raise the standards of service provided by workers and to instill confidence, goodwill, and understanding among the membership and their employers toward the end of preventing unnecessary conflicts or serious misunderstandings.
- To establish a spirit of cooperation, good faith, and fair dealings with all employers, and to secure for its membership reasonable hours, fair wages, and improved working conditions through the process of collective bargaining.
- To initiate and promote such legislation as may be for the best interests of the members of this organization.
- To protect the rights of workers and the welfare of its members through political, educational, and legislative activity; to engage in cultural, civic legislative, political, fraternal, educational, social, and other activities that further the interests of the organization and its members and/or improve their standing in the community.

- To safeguard, advance, and promote the principle of free collective bargaining in a democratic society.
- To protect and preserve the right of this organization to perform its legal and contractual obligations and to carry out the duties and responsibilities entrusted to it by the membership.
- To promote the economic and social welfare of the members of this organization through unity of action and mutual cooperation (American Federation of Teachers).

Elder suggests that most problems stem from middle managers who are made to enforce rules created by upper management. He believes collective bargaining organizations eliminate conflict that is inherent with middle managers trying to please upper management while putting employees at risk. Elder says, "A good manager is not threatened by a union, and is glad to have a contract. . . . A good manager can still communicate, encourage, and motivate employees with a collective bargaining contract (telephone interview, 7 June 1998).

Elder believes that there is safety in numbers and that nurses as well as other workers have more clout against unfair management practices than the individual does. Collective bargaining provides power to the front-line workers and defines what it is that workers owe to their employer.

Collective bargaining organizations also provide education and information to members and representatives about effective collective bargaining strategies. Guidelines exist for evaluating employees, facilitating negotiations, negotiating contracts, dealing with employee grievances, and mediating employee-employer disputes. For their membership dues, each member receives supplemental information, a copy of the union contract, and ongoing communication.

Collective bargaining organizations charge a monthly stipend for members, usually deducted from paychecks. Dues can cost anywhere from 200 to 900 dollars per year. Newsletters and ongoing communication on relevant collective bargaining issues, pending legislation, policy changes, and other information are provided to members regularly. Telephone hotlines are set up to provide information on an urgent basis to members or to disperse information on a specific issue, such as an impending strike.

It is the perception of union negotiators that "nothing is more important to the effectiveness of a labor organization than unity guided by intelligence" (Kaysee Rowlett, memorandum, 1989). Rowlett writes, "Unless a union acts together, concentrating its strength and directing its efforts towards common goals, it will not be effective in obtaining better wages and benefits nor in establishing harmonious working conditions with respect and dignity on the job for all employees." According to Rowlett:

> Nothing is more destructive of unity than the absence of agency shop provisions from a collective bargaining agreement. Unions represent all members of the bargaining units, including those who are not members. More importantly, such representation promotes unity and therefore strengthens the union and its ability to obtain improved working conditions. When a collective bargaining agreement lacks agency shop provisions, bargaining unit members who have not joined the union benefit from the union's efforts equally with members, but do not pay their fair share of the cost of obtaining such benefits. In other words, non-members get a "free ride." Professional representation costs money. Without agency shops, free-riders could seriously undermine the union's ability to perform its representational functions. The legislature has provided a remedy for the unfairness of open shops called "organizational security" (1989).

## UNION SECURITY

Unions were able to create union security clauses through legislation passed beginning in 1935. The National Labor Relations Board (NLRB) Act of 1935 was established to protect the right to strong unions. Consequently, it permitted high union security. There are several types of union security:

- *Closed shop*—This means that an employer and a union could create an agreement under which the employer agreed to hire and retain only persons who were members of the union. The NLRB Act was amended in 1947 to expressly prohibit closed shops.
- *Union shop*—The strictest form of union security permitted under the revised law is the union shop. An employer must hire without regard to union membership. However, a union shop clause can require an employee to join the union after a grace period and to remain a union

member during the agreement. The grace period must be at least 30 days.

- *Agency shop*—This clause does not require a covered employee to become a union member, but does require the employee to pay the union a fee for the services and benefits accruing to the employee because of the union. These fees can legally be equivalent in amount to the initiation fees and dues paid by full union members.
- *Objector option agency shop*—Employees may opt out of agency shop requirements provided they are employed prior to a dated stated in the union contract and not members on that date. Employees may exercise a one-time option for exemption from agency shop by filing timely written objections with both the union and the employer.
- *Modified agency shop*—All employees who come into the bargaining unit after a date stated in the agreement shall either join the union or pay service fees to the union for the duration of the contract.
- *Maintenance of membership*—A maintenance of membership clause does not require an employee to join a union or to pay a service fee. Instead, it requires an employee who has voluntarily become a member of the union to remain a member. It is not unusual to find a collective bargaining agreement containing two union security clauses: a union shop clause covering all new hires and a maintenance of membership clause for those employed prior to the signing of the contract establishing the union shop.
- *Open shop*—Where there is no negotiated union security agreement, the labor-management relationship is referred to as an open shop. The union is legally bound to represent all workers in the bargaining unit, but workers are not required to be union members.

Employees are also allowed exemption on religious grounds from joining a union, and this exemption is protected by law. Unions may also use hiring halls. Hiring halls are employment offices conducted by a union to secure jobs for members and provide referrals to employers. Hiring halls are frequently confused with closed shops. Although the two are linked historically, they are not the same. A hiring hall arrangement under which an employer agrees to hire through the union is not unlawful if it does not discriminate against applicants with regard to their membership or nonmembership in the union. However, a union may charge nonmembers a service fee to help pay expenses. The service fee cannot be equal to dues because it would create a union shop. The hiring hall provision can operate in conjunction with a union shop clause so that all workers, whether members or not, may be required to become members after the grace period.

A portion of the Taft-Hartley Act, Section 14b, permits individual states to outlaw the negotiation of union security clauses. This means states may pass laws prohibiting collective bargaining agreements that make union membership a condition of continuing employment. Such laws create the compulsory open shop in which the union must represent everyone in the bargaining unit but no one is compelled to belong to the union. There are 21 states that have right to work laws.

Under present law, a union shop clause negotiated by a union with majority status is presumed valid. However, upon petition of 30 percent of the employees in a unit, the NLRB will conduct a deauthorization election to determine whether a majority desires to rescind the union's authorization to apply a union security agreement. In a deauthorization election, a majority of employees in a unit, as opposed to a majority of those voting, must vote to rescind the union's authority. If the deauthorization is successful, the NLRB will immediately declare the existing union security provision invalid.

## THE PRO-UNION POSITION

There are both pro and con arguments about unionization and organizational security issues. Individuals favoring unions believe they represent employees who are unable to represent themselves successfully. This is not totally unlike the advocacy role that nursing takes on to represent patients who are unable to represent themselves. Pro-union folks believe that employees require assistance with workplace issues and could not achieve individually what can be achieved by the masses. Unions provide updates on current issues (such as OSHA regulations) and help secure legislation that protects employees (such as the Violence in the Workplace Act, enacted in 1997).

Union supporters suggest that collective bargaining organizations are focused on the approach of mutual gains, problem solving, and bargaining relationships. In his article in *CASBO Journal* on union negotiating, George Jeffers suggests that unions that use the following strategies as operating principles will be successful:

- Develop an agreed-on problem statement for both parties.
- Explore both parties' interests in settling issues on the table.
- Examine each party's alternatives for settlement.
- Create settlement options for both parties to use together.
- Define criteria for validation of settlement options.
- Communicate openly with each other.
- Develop a trusting, committed relationship (Jeffers, 1997).

Probably most important from the unions' perspective is the fact that collective bargaining agreements permit consolidation of the union position as representatives of a bargaining unit. Organizational security clauses are beneficial because the union is freed from continuous organizing activity directed at maintaining its majority status and representation rights among the employees in a unit. New employees routinely become members, the employer is stripped of the ability to woo employees away from the union, other unions are discouraged from raiding the unit, and the unions' bargaining position is strengthened.

In terms of public interest, employer-union agreements tend to promote long-term relationships. Such agreements can also minimize conflict, especially between workers, where conflict often arises around job expectations, salaries, or benefits. In addition, these agreements eliminate the potential conflicts likely to arise when members work alongside workers who are not union members.

## THE ANTI-UNION POSITION

Those who do not support the concept of union representation argue that unions are not needed if management and employees keep communication open and work together from a perspective of honesty and mutual support. Others argue that individuals are forced to join unions because of contract and specific shop clauses. These may deprive those individuals who do not want to join or support a union of the opportunity to obtain and keep a job in a workplace with union representation.

Union naysayers also claim that employee-union relationships are no more than a financial obligation to self-serving individuals who want to control the workplace. These folks believe that unions collect dues which are little more than the purchase price of benefits and privileges of a union contract that could be obtained without the collective strength provided by union membership.

Health care associations representing employers and health care providers are the biggest union opponents. They often support legislation that weakens union influence and retains employer control of provider services. These associations often prepare information for provider members outlining principles that health care facilities should follow in order to minimize union receptivity among employees.

Managers and supervisors need to be trained to oversee the work of others and be granted the authority by senior management to function effectively. Clear supervisory authority, backed by policies and procedures, can usually minimize employee–management conflict. Clearly delineated grievance and problem-solving procedures also clarify to employees that management is interested in resolving conflict, not ignoring it.

## UNION ACTIVITY IN THE WORKPLACE

The circumstances that motivate employees to seek union assistance usually arise from inadequate communication between management and employees or an employee perception of poor treatment by management. Occasionally, payment/benefits issues or job insecurity can also trigger employee interest in union representation. It is a well-known rule in health care management that employees who are unhappy are more likely to seek union support and contact labor representation.

Many health care facilities dealing with managed care delivery have faced almost all of these issues in the 1990s. Health care facilities are often counseled by labor relations experts that there are early warning signs to watch for *before* unions are actually voted in that indicate union organizing may be occurring.

Employees have looked to unions for help when problems arise in the workplace. Unfortunately, many employees do not understand that although union representation can resolve some employer-related problems, it also introduces new issues and costs—such as dues or fines—as well as new issues—such as strikes and crossing picket lines. For nurses, union representation remains a complex issue.

## UNIONS AND HEALTH CARE

Unions are a powerful force in health care. It is unclear if they will maintain this influence over time. Elder believes that it is time for industry to "sit up and take notice" of unions and their value to employees. He also believes that there is a point where either the union or the employers can become too powerful, and that that is not useful to either group.

Unions will continue to use the media to send their message. Media exposure was a successful strategy for the UPS strike in 1998. Health care providers are concerned about their image in the public eye, and strikes do not improve public image. Kaiser has had to deal with a great deal of media coverage of its ongoing issues with the California Nurses Association, which has made bargaining more difficult, led other organizations to be more leery of union activity, and often made Kaiser appear greedy and power hungry.

As an author and a nurse, it has been a struggle to write a balanced chapter on unions. It is my personal belief that unions do not benefit—and in fact demean—the profession of nursing. However, as long as employees believe their dignity and value are threatened, unions will remain powerful. If health care providers come to grips with how they are dealing with employees, restructuring, and the constantly changing health care environment, unions will not be so attractive to employees. Each nurse must decide for herself or himself the value of unionization in the professional nursing role. Research the unions representing nurses in your local area and learn how they have dealt with health care issues. Only then can you determine the best decision for your professional practice.

## DISCUSSION QUESTIONS

1. Are nurses represented by collective bargaining organizations in your local area? Why or why not?
2. Are unions good or bad for the professional role of nursing? Why?
3. What strategies do unions use to organize successfully in your local area?
4. What could health care providers do differently to discourage union activity, if anything?
5. Is there union activity in your state? Why?

**BIBLIOGRAPHY**

American Association of Critical-Care Nurses. 1996. "Decision Grid for Delegation." Staffing Tool Kit. Aliso Viejo, California: AACN Publishing.

American Federation of Teachers

American Nurses' Association. 1985. *Code for Nurses*. Washington, D.C.: ANA Publishing.

———. 1993. *Nursing's Agenda for Health Care Reform*. Washington, D.C.: ANA Publishing.

———. 1994. *Every Patient Deserves a Nurse*. Brochure. Washington, D.C.: ANA Publishing.

———. 1995. *Nursing's Social Policy Statement*. Washington, D.C.: ANA Publishing.

———. 1996a. *Registered Professional Nurses and Unlicensed Assistive Personnel*. 2nd ed. Washington, D.C.: ANA Publishing.

———. 1996b. *Scope and Standards of Advanced Practice Registered Nursing*. Washington, D.C.: ANA Publishing.

American Organization of Nurse Executives. 1996. *Talking Points on Hospital Redesign*. Washington, D.C.: American Organization of Nurse Executives.

Burda, D. 1994. "Layoffs Rise as Pace of Cost-Cutting Accelerates." *Modern Healthcare*, 12 December, 32.

———. 1995. "ANA Report Stokes Restructuring Debate." *Modern Healthcare*, 13 February, 38.

California Healthcare Association. 1990. "Unions." Handouts/lecture materials, May 1990. Oxnard, California.

California Nurses Association. Web Site Home Page. http://www.califnurses.org/

California Taxpayers Against Higher Health Costs. 1996. Ballot materials.

Izzo, J. 1998. "The Changing Values of Workers." *Healthcare Forum Journal*, May/June, 62–65.

Jeffers, G. 1997. "Achieving Closure in Interest-Based Bargaining." *CASBO Journal* (fall), 19–25.

Kunen, J. 1996. "The New Hands-Off Nursing." *Time*, 30 September, 55–57.

Lumsdon, K.. 1995. "Faded Glory." *Hospitals and Health Networks*, 5 December, 31–36.

Malone, B. et al. 1996. "A Grim Prognosis for Healthcare." *American Journal of Nursing Survey Results*, November, 40.

Moore, J.D. Jr. 1997. "Sunshine on Kaiser Data." *Modern Healthcare,* 10 November, 52.


National Council of Nursing State Boards. 1995. "Delegation." *Issues 95* 15(1): 1–3.

Olmos, D. 1997. "HMO Panel to Call for Consumer Protections." *Los Angeles Times*, 31 December, 1.

Organization of Nurse Leaders. 1995. "Focus Group Notes." *Nursing Issues,* 29 September.

Rowlett, K. 1996. American Federation of Teachers. Memoranda to union members and representatives.

Sherer, J. 1994a. "Job Shifts." *Hospitals and Health Networks*, 5 October, 64–68.

———. 1994b. "Union Uprising: California Nurses React Aggressively to Work Redesign." *Hospitals and Health Networks*, 20 December, 36–38.

Shindul-Rothschild, J. et al. 1997. "Ten Keys to Quality Care." *American Journal of Nursing* 97(11): 35–43.

Shubert, D. 1996. "Hospitals Decrease Nurses' Role: Reassign Tasks to Aides." *Los Angeles Times*, 14 July.

Turner, S.O. 1995. "Reality Check: It's Time for Nursing to Face the Future." *Hospitals and Health Networks*, 20 August, 20–22.

# CHAPTER 17

# Thriving in the New Environment

> This chapter presents several different strategies for dealing with situations, events, and people—including yourself. All are aimed at providing today's nurse with the skills and mindset to thrive in the managed care marketplace.

## USING YOUR EMOTIONAL INTELLIGENCE TO ENHANCE YOUR CAREER*

A few years ago, a new concept about intelligence was identified in the marketplace. Emotional intelligence, a new way to consider intellectual ability, embodied an entirely different theoretical framework for evaluating individuals' successes and abilities.

It used to be that business success was determined solely on the basis of facts and numbers. However, the bottom line is that every purchase, whatever the product or service, involves emotions.

This fuzzy, interpersonal side of the workplace now has a name, emotional intelligence. The concept of emotional intelligence was first developed by Peter Salovey and John Mayer. It was popularized by Daniel Goleman, who wrote *Emotional Intelligence: Why It Can Matter More Than IQ* (1995). The subject has received a lot of attention because it is the first attempt to quantify people's emotions and interpersonal reactions.

---

*Source: Courtesy of Hendrie Weisinger, Westport, Connecticut.

227

An emotional quotient (EQ), like an intelligence quotient (IQ), is multi-faceted. It is more than common sense. Different emotional qualities, from how we handle anger or face failure to how approachable we seem to others, apply to every part of our business lives. In many cases, a high EQ matters more than a high IQ (Beakley, 1998).

For some, the qualities that compose a high emotional intelligence seem common-sense based: Be nice to people, don't make decisions when you are angry, etc. But EQ goes beyond niceness, or even morality. It is a measurable set of skills, like driving or typing, although much more complex. Like other skills, EQ can be improved and enhanced.

Nurses have been using their "gut instinct" to survive in the workplace. Nurses are usually quite good at assessing and evaluating the emotional state of others. This awareness has always proved useful to nurses, but there has never been any theoretical framework to support this practice. Now nurses can understand why it is beneficial. In the words of one manager, IQ gets you hired, but EQ gets you promoted.

### Components of Emotional Intelligence

Hendrie Weisinger, PhD, is one of the nation's leading experts in emotional intelligence. It is his view that emotional intelligence is far more important in determining workplace success than traditional IQ ratings of intellectual capability. Dr. Weisinger defined emotional intelligence as a collection of abilities (1998). Those abilities, when enhanced, can offer improved chances for success in the workplace. The collection of abilities Dr. Weisinger defines as emotional intelligence include four key abilities, as well as key personality factors that enhance emotional intelligence.

1. The ability to perceive accurately, appraise, and express emotion.

This means that an individual can accurately understand and evaluate her own emotions, as well as express them. In addition, this individual can also assess and interpret emotions expressed by others. Nurses are particularly good at using this ability because they are trained to observe and assess the behavior of patients.

2. The ability to access and/or generate feelings when they facilitate thought.

In addition to this second, key ability, an individual must possess empathy and be in tune to others' feelings and perceptions. Individuals with strong emotional intelligence are able to use their own past experiences to relate to the circumstances and feelings of others. Nurses are skilled in this area also, as many nurses have the ability to share and understand feelings with their patients. Dr. Weisinger points out that oftentimes when an individual demonstrates anxiety at work, that person is really feeling uncertainty. The ability to empathize with this emotion and the behaviors it provokes rather than become defensive is crucial to relating well to co-workers.

3. The ability to understand emotion and to have emotional knowledge.

This means that individuals can articulate to themselves and others what emotions are trying to tell them. Weisinger believes that all emotions are intrinsically good and they transcend time and culture. Individuals skilled in emotional intelligence have the ability to intellectually understand what their emotions mean and why those particular emotions are occurring. Nurses are usually pretty good at observing and articulating the emotions of patients, but not as good at assessing and articulating their own emotions and their meaning. Nurses also tend to label emotions as "good" or "bad," which causes judgment to occur.

4. The ability to regulate emotions to promote emotional and intellectual growth.

Dr. Weisinger believes that to be successful in the workplace, an individual must be able to turn on or restrain emotions appropriately, as if on cue. He believes that in the workplace, all workers need emotion management and self-motivation to manage their own emotions in order to be successful. In other words, an individual cannot let her emotions get the better of her in the workplace.

### Positive Denial

It takes self-control and self-motivation to skillfully control emotions in the work setting. Weisinger believes the most critical skill for managing emotions is that of positive denial. Positive denial means that an individual is able to deal with an issue, but at a distance, with a buffer. The person can step back and "deal with it tomorrow," and then deal with the issue in smaller, incremental steps. Nurses are not particularly adept at this skill, either. Perhaps due to inability to handle conflict well, or simply because some emotions are difficult to manage, nurses are not usually able to buffer their own feelings or those of others. Instead, in many cases, the feelings are "buried" or completely denied, often with the use of alcohol or drugs to deaden the intensity of the feelings.

### Self-Awareness

Dr. Weisinger believes that high self-awareness is a critical factor in successfully using emotional intelligence. High self-awareness refers to having an accurate understanding of how you behave and how other people perceive you, recognizing how you respond to others, being sensitive to your attitudes, feelings, emotions, intentions, and general communication style at any given moment, and being able to accurately disclose this awareness to others (Weisinger, 1998).

Some skill indicators of the self-awareness factor include knowing when you are thinking negatively, becoming angry, becoming defensive, or experiencing a mood shift. In addition, Weisinger believes you must know how you are interpreting events you encounter and what senses you are using to do so, be able to accurately communicate what you are experiencing, and know the impact that your behavior has on others. These are skills for use in the workplace. Nurses tend to be great at using these skills to accurately assess patients, but may be less able to assess themselves.

Ways to assess your self-awareness include answering questions such as:

- Do I recognize my feelings and emotions as they happen?
- Am I aware of how others perceive me?
- How do I act when I am defensive?
- Am I aware of how I speak to myself?
- Am I aware of my organization's needs?

Dr. Weisinger's tips for developing high self-awareness include:

- Examine how you make appraisals.
- Tune in to your senses.
- Get in touch with your feelings.
- Learn what your intentions are.
- Pay attention to your actions.

### Managing Emotions

Another critical success factor in using emotional intelligence in the workplace is the ability to manage emotions, according to Dr. Weisinger (1998). Managing emotions is the capacity to soothe oneself, to shake off rampant anxiety, gloom, or irritability; and to be able to keep emotional perspective. Some of the skill indicators of this factor include being able to identify shifts in physiological arousal, act productively in anger- or anxiety-producing situations, calm oneself quickly when angry, associate different physiological cues with different emotional states, and use internal speech to affect emotional states and status.

Ways to assess the way you manage emotions include answering these questions:

- Do I use anger productively?
- Can I manage my anxiety in times of change?
- Can I put myself in a good mood?
- Do I think that asking others for help is a sign of weakness?

From a psychological perspective, there are three components of the emotional system. First is the cognitive emotion—how you feel. Second is physical arousal—how your body responds to how you feel. Third is the behavior you exhibit based on the other two components. All three of these components must be managed for you to be successful in the workplace. I would venture to guess that most nurses (including this one) need some work in this area!

Tips for managing your emotions, according to Dr. Weisinger, include:

- Use your thoughts as instructional self-statements to keep you on track.
- Avoid distorted thinking.
- Use relaxation techniques to decrease your physical arousal.
- Become a good problem solver by focusing on situation.
- Recognize that problems are actually your poor response to the situation.
- Use and generate humor.
- Take time out; recognize that when you are frustrated, angry, or defensive you will be a poor problem solver or situation-responder!

### *Self-Motivation*

Another factor that Dr. Weisinger believes is critical for successfully using emotional intelligence is the ability to motivate oneself. Motivating oneself is defined as being able to channel emotions to achieve a goal. This includes being able to postpone immediate gratification for future gratification, being productive in low-interest activities, being able to persist in the face of frustration, and being able to generate initiation without the influence of external factors.

Skill indicators identified by Dr. Weisinger for this factor include being able to gear up at will, regroup quickly after a setback, complete long-term tasks in designated time frames, and produce high energy when doing un-interesting or low-enjoyment work. In addition, other skill indicators are the ability to change and stop ineffective habits, develop new and produc-tive behavior patterns, and follow through on words with actions.

Individuals can assess their level of self-motivation by asking:

- Am I persistent?
- Do setbacks set me back?
- Can I psych myself up?

Dr. Weisinger's tips for self-motivation (getting yourself to do some-thing) include:

- Use all sources of motivation.
- Play mental games.
- Use a support system.
- Keep tasks "underwhelming."
- Make your environment task-friendly.
- Utilize emotional arousal for energy.

### Interpersonal Expertise

Another factor Dr. Weisinger considers important for emotional intelli-gence success is interpersonal expertise. Interpersonal expertise means being able to exchange information on a meaningful level and includes the skills necessary for organizing groups and building teams, negotiating so-lutions, mediating conflict among others, building consensus and making personal connections.

Skill indicators for this factor include being able to use effective inter-personal communication techniques, influence others directly or indi-rectly, articulate the thoughts of a group, build trust, and make others feel good. Individuals with these skills are often sought out by others for advice and support.

Tips for assessing your interpersonal effectiveness, according to Dr. Weisinger, include asking yourself these questions:

- Is it easy for me to resolve conflicts?
- How well do I give criticism?
- Am I a good listener?
- Do I frequently praise people?

## *Communication*

Interpersonal expertise in the workplace means how good you are at helping others by listening and working with a team. Interpersonal expertise involves different levels of communication including passing communication (sharing information), factual information (writing letters or memos), and thoughts, ideas, and feelings. Key communication skills have been identified as being crucial to many dimensions of interpersonal effectiveness, including leadership, management, and working well with others. The key communication skills for using emotional intelligence are:

- Self-disclosure
- Dynamic listening
- Assertiveness
- Criticism
- Problem solving
- Team skills

Dr. Weisinger believes that emotional intelligence can be blended into communication. Tips for using this strategy include using sensitivity, being aware of your own personal "filters," being tuned into the emotional subtext, and assessing your risk of self-disclosure. Tips for developing interpersonal expertise by blending emotional intelligence into communication include:

- Analyze the relationship (boundaries, expectations, perceptions, encounters).
- Communicate at the appropriate information exchange level.

## *Emotional Mentoring*

The last factor involving successful use of emotional intelligence in the workplace is emotional mentoring of others. Emotional mentoring of others is defined as being aware of other people's feelings and emotions (it is *not* feeling responsible for them!), being able to listen to their feelings, being able to help others deal with their feelings and emotions in productive ways, and assisting others in increasing their awareness about their current affective state.

Dr. Weisinger's skill indicators for this factor include being able to accurately reflect back to others the feelings they are experiencing, stay calm in the presence of others' distressful emotions, recognize when others are distressed, and help others manage their emotions. In addition, other skill indicators include being perceived as empathic and having the ability to engage in intimate conversations with others, manage group emotions, and detect incongruences between others' emotions and feelings and their behavior.

Tips for assessing how you manage the emotions and feelings of others include asking these questions of yourself:

- Am I skillful in managing the emotions of others?
- How do I know when my boss or colleagues are angry, sad, anxious, etc.?
- Can I manage an angry group?
- Am I comfortable with my feelings?

While nurses are exceptionally good at observing and assessing others' emotions and feelings, many nurses struggle with a sense of responsibility for fixing others' emotional states.

Dr. Weisinger's tips for emotional mentoring (Weisinger, 1998) include:

- Keep your emotional perspective.
- Calm the out-of-control person.
- Use supportive listening.
- Help with goal planning and achievement.

Although using emotional intelligence, applying communication skills, and providing emotional mentoring of others may seem unrelated to dealing with managed care and far from the main focus of this book, I believe that nurses who use emotional intelligence skills at work will be more successful in this tumultuous health care environment and happier than those who don't.

## SELF-EMPOWERMENT TO THRIVE IN MANAGED CARE[*]

Are you a self-empowered person? Marilyn Murray Willison completed an unofficial study of the lives of self-empowered women and discovered they share 17 traits in common. While the author recognizes the study data

---

[*]*Source:* Written by J. Oldham. Copyright, *Los Angeles Times*. Reprinted by permission.

is only relevant to females, all readers are encouraged to assess the information and apply it to their own personal situation, regardless of gender.

Initially, Willison started noticing a pattern in the lives of self-empowered women. Whether they were black or white, young or old, scientist or artist, was secondary. In spite of their apparent differences, these self-empowered women all seemed to share a startling number of characteristics. Willison started cataloging successful women, researching their lives and comparing the patterns that kept reappearing. The same traits and attitudes came up over and over. Time after time, the self-empowering scenario repeated itself until, after Willison had learned one snippet of information about an ambitious woman's life, she could actually begin to predict what would happen next.

What she learned is that there are reasons why some women make it and others don't. Women who are true achievers share many of the same traits, and these common characteristics actually take some of the "magic" out of their success. These are ordinary women who simply have goals and attitudes—rather than gifts or advantages—that far surpass the ordinary. Successful women have an attitude, an approach to their future that sets them apart from other women. There are plenty of well educated, well connected women who have not achieved their goals and may be confused about why. However, in Willison's opinion, success is not an accident. Certain women get on the fast track and stay there. Here's how.

1. Nonexistent Paternal Safety Net. One trait that shows up again and again with achieving women is the fact that they tend to learn early in life to depend upon themselves and not rely on their father. Therefore, they are forced to develop a lifelong habit of looking within for what they want and need out of life.
2. Early Sense of Direction. Most high-achieving women know what they want to do with their lives prior to being shaped by the cultural limitations of being female. They envisioned limitless horizons and possibilities. By the time these girls encountered the issues of femininity that have detoured many promising careers, they had already decided exactly how they wanted their lives to progress.
3. Believe in the Unbelievable. Many of these women in their youth were exposed to someone who was either intensely religious or spiritual. While this exposure to belief did not inspire these women as girls to necessarily become religious themselves, it did impress

upon them the need to structure one's life around and believing in something that cannot be seen or proven. The exposure to this devout belief can be from anyone, but what matters is that the child sees someone older who commits him or herself to an invisible power. While women are still in the struggling stages, learning to operate on faith is sometimes the only way to become a true convert to the cause of our future success.

4. The Significant Other. These women all had someone who stood out as a pivotal force in helping make the dream come true. Each woman found someone who reinforced her self-image and supported her later development. The role the significant other played was to reflect back to us the picture of ourselves that keeps us striving toward a goal.

5. Life Is Not a Popularity Contest. Women who achieve their life goals seem to recognize that being popular isn't important.

6. Life Is Not a Beauty Pageant. The women Willison studied were more often than not strong and attractive. However, the women rarely saw themselves that way. They developed a habit of thinking in terms of what they did rather than how they looked.

7. The Magnificent Obsession. The women Willison studied had a remarkable sense of tenacity when it came to their chosen goals. Even when they received little reinforcement from the world at large, they were able to keep plugging away at their dreams.

8. Turning No into Yes. The achievers studied by Willison all heard plenty of negative remarks during their long journey to success. Where most of us would be crippled by implied rejection of turndowns, their women instinctively used the "no" to either improve their work or spur them on to greater achievement. These women seem to realize that "no" was an opinion rather than a fact.

9. Music. Willison was surprised to discover that many of the self-empowered women she studied shared a deep sense of music appreciation. Even when these achievers did not play a musical instrument themselves, music still spoke to them in a special moving way.

10. The Critic Within. Most of the women researched were fortunate enough to rely on themselves for motivation. In addition, Willison found they had the advantage of consistent, self-generated criticism. These women seemed to rely on themselves to judge and refine and improve rather than wait for others to tell them what was right or wrong.

11. Risk Addiction. These women who have reached their goals all seemed to train themselves not only to cope well but to hunger for pressure. They were able to deal with unexpected opportunities that involved risk, and turn difficult situations into ones that enhanced their futures. There is a clear-cut behavior pattern of not only not attempting to avoid risk, but welcoming it.

12. Hard Times. Very few of the successful women Willison studied were "overnight" successes. The road was invariably a long tortuous one. Many of the women faced strikingly demoralizing circumstances before they had any reward or success.

13. More Than Meets the Eye. Many of these successful women had to cope with having other people chronically underestimate their abilities. Often, they were treated in patronizing or diminishing ways. Fortunately, these women held on to their own vision of the future rather than buy into other people's perceptions.

14. Selective Disassociation. One unusual aspect that Willison found successful women share is the power to selectively disassociate themselves from people, places, and things that might interfere with the fulfillment of their dreams. This aloofness seems to help these achievers move ever onward instead of staying mired among safe, familiar surroundings.

15. Forget about Prince Charming. Willison found that many self-empowered women have turbulent love lives. Many struggled with numerous unsatisfying relationships, marriages, and divorce before finding supportive partners.

16. Motherhood. Willison also noted that these self-empowered and over-achieving women take their motherhood role seriously. They are ferociously devoted to their children and consider motherhood a special fulfillment.

17. Dreaming Your Own Dream. These women focus their energies and ambitions on themselves. They rarely absorb other people's goals and don't try to impress their aspirations on other people. They refuse to fill the expectations that other people have for their futures. It takes strength, vision, and courage to fulfill your own dreams, particularly if they are in opposition to the desires of those we love.

\* \* \* \*

*A note from the author:* The purpose for including these traits in a book for nurses on managed care is because nurses must become self-empowered. Learning how to get what you want out of life is not a gift given to you by someone else. It is a skill that can be learned and cultivated. Anyone who wants to can intentionally acquire the traits discussed here—traits that the self-empowered women studied by Willison learned accidentally.

## BEING GRACIOUS IS MANDATORY!

We have all been on the receiving end of a "networking nightmare": a time when someone was rude to us at a meeting, didn't follow through as expected or promised, or took unfair advantage of our professional contacts. Even though you may go through downsizing, layoffs, mergers, or other difficult career experiences, rude behavior and unprofessional etiquette have no place in the work setting. Be sure your graciousness is up to par.

When introduced to someone, say hello and make eye contact. Try to avoid scanning nametags in a room of people for the purpose of cultivating those who will be useful to you and skipping over those whose job titles don't interest you. Be sure your attitude is not "How can you help me?" Make sure you meet someone because of inviting eye contact, not because you are shopping for important people. Don't drone on with self-importance when introducing yourself. And try not to give someone your title as if it is explanation enough of who you are. Try practicing a 15-second introduction of who you are and what you do.

After meeting a new colleague or making a promise of assistance, you should send a note or leave a follow-through voice mail message within 10 days. To make someone wait longer to hear from you, or to fail to make contact at all, is sloppy and unprofessional. Develop a system to deal with the business cards you get so that they are not misplaced or forgotten. Try writing note on the backs of business cards to help you remember who the persons are and where you met them, as well as any promise you made to them to follow-up.

Do you listen when people talk with you? If you continually find yourself asking a question twice because you didn't catch the answer the first time, you may need to improve your listening skills. If you are bored with a conversation, you might finish a comment, smile, and politely say, "Excuse me, it was nice meeting you. I see my boss. . . . " Then be sure to move to a different area in the room and begin another conversation with someone else.

Make sure you are seen as a giver in your community. Be certain your name shows up at industry functions as either a donor or a doer. By joining professional organizations, you will build a reputation as someone who is serious about your profession, career, and contacts. Don't wait for a crisis to start professional networking. Many people wait for a major change in their job status—layoff, relocation, or termination—and then scramble around in a panic asking themselves, "Who do I know?" Make sure you build a group of contacts when things are going well for you. Then, when you do need help, you will have people to call on.

Make sure you interact with younger and less experienced professionals as well. Most people want to interact only with those who are successful, but it is also important to interact and mentor those just starting out. Since health care and nursing are very close knit industries, someone you mentor today could be your superior in a few years!

Take the time to write a thank-you note or call when someone has helped you. It is crucial to be perceived as gracious. In addition, doing so sends the message that you are not just a taker, and it makes people want to help you again.

## NETWORKING: A METHOD TO CREATE CONNECTIONS

Networking is the process of creating linkages to obtain information, influence, and power. It is the process of exchanging information between strategically placed individuals who have access to ideas and other people. Networking is a process of developing and using contacts to assist you in accomplishing your goals, solving problems, and advancing your career.

Networking is a critical business skill and component to a successful career. Networking can be done in social situations with family and friends or at focused business meetings. Effective networking requires a conscious commitment of time, energy, and resources. It is a long-term strategy for professional and career advancement. The rewards are rarely immediate and the benefits sometimes take years to be realized.

Networking is an active process and cannot be accomplished by default. Time must be scheduled and dedicated to contacting and connecting with colleagues. Networking is *not* calling colleagues only when you need something. It is actively managing professional relationships to mutually benefit both parties and advance both of your careers.

Professional networking includes activities such as making phone calls just to chat. These calls are important even when you don't need anything.

Contact colleagues to share information on open positions, industry news, and the like. When you are contacted by a colleague, promptly return phone calls with the information requested.

If a colleague assists you with a contact or referral, write a thank-you note. It is considered not only gracious but mandatory professional etiquette to say thank you for favors received from colleagues.

You can phone colleagues to ask for assistance with solving a problem or developing a new program. This allows you to gain valuable information on a project without having to "reinvent the wheel." You can also receive potential job referrals or business contacts that may result in future work relationships.

The networking method I use most frequently is to take colleagues and potential network contacts out for lunch. Because I am self-employed and work out of my home, I must create networking activities that keep me in touch with potential clients, existing clients, and valuable colleagues.

Networking can help you accomplish your professional goals. First, identify your personal career goals. Then, identify the existing networks available, and those most appropriate to achieve your goals. These networks may be personal colleagues or professional nursing specialty organizations.

It is important to initiate contacts within the most appropriate networks. You need to cultivate the contacts you make, keeping in touch on a regular basis. You can also use those contacts for career advancement. Call these colleagues when you are considering changing jobs or taking a promotion. They can provide important data about the industry in general, and an objective "outsider" view on issues within your own facility.

Successful strategies for professional networking include routinely contacting colleagues in other local facilities. These can be nurses in roles such as yours, or in roles that you might want in the future. It is also helpful to subscribe to at least one motivational or business magazine. It does not have to be a nursing journal; in fact, a general business magazine may be most useful.

Try to develop one important local business contact. Initiate and maintain that contact through phone calls and regular meetings. The meetings can be social, such as meeting for lunch, dinner, or drinks, and do not have to be frequent. Meeting for dinner once or twice a year with a trusted colleague can be extremely valuable to your career.

Invest in yourself and your future by participating in educational opportunities (that is, go back to school to get your BSN), specialized programs, and subscriptions. Become active and visible in your local nursing community. This provides numerous networking opportunities in the local area.

You will also need to learn specific networking behaviors. Develop a firm handshake and strong eye contact with strangers. Learn to write thank-you notes to everyone who did a favor for you or gave you a valuable contact. You must also develop good listening and communication skills to allow you to be a valuable networking colleague for other nurses. *Never* burn your bridges by gossiping or becoming mistrusted with professional confidences. This will cause you to be avoided as a networking professional.

Mentoring is also a valuable networking strategy. It is extremely underutilized in nursing. In fact, nurses tend to "eat their young" and not professionally mentor new nurses. Mentoring is a process where a seasoned executive takes an inexperienced person "under his or her wing" and shows the newcomer "the ropes." It can be formal or informal.

Mentors serve as teachers, sponsors/references, hosts, role models, and counselors. If you have a difficult situation in your present job or role, you can discuss the problem with your mentors and ask for suggestions. If you are considering changing jobs or advancing your education, mentors are great to bounce ideas off of.

Nurses need to learn the mentorship role. Most nurses have not been exposed to good mentorship models. Mentorship is not about power. It is about facilitating and helping other nurses. Mentoring is not dependent on education or roles. I have two very special mentors in my professional life. One is a master's-prepared nurse executive I met while in graduate school. The other is a diploma school graduate with 33 years of registered nursing experience, primarily in the ER. She showed me the ropes as a nursing student and still continues to have a strong effect on my professional decisions.

## SHOULD YOU MOVE INTO A NURSING MANAGEMENT ROLE?

If you are considering moving into nursing management and climbing the organizational ladder, there are some issues to consider.

Are you willing to get additional training? Expanding your job-related education is an effective way to move ahead. Obtaining a degree isn't always necessary, but acquiring essential skills sets definitely is. Employers are looking for excellent written and oral communication and an ability to effectively manage staff and workloads. According to Robin Ryan, author of *24 Hours to Your Next Job, Raise or Promotion (1997)*, to increase your chances of promotion, take classes that focus on supervision and communication skills. There are national programs that offer one-day seminars, and your local college is another possible resource.

Are you able to coach others? The ability to motivate others and oversee their work is critical in nursing. If you are a computer ace, offer to train co-workers, even if it is not part of your present job description. This will provide supervisory experience beyond the scope of your job. Whenever possible, volunteer to oversee per diem or registry staff, or head up a committee or project. Make sure that you know how to give clear directions and to tactfully check to see that the work is progressing correctly and in a timely manner. Evaluate your awareness that there are multiple ways to get a job done effectively, and polish your ability to encourage people.

Can you make decisions and delegate? Both are key functions of managers. Managers must assign tasks, plan projects, and make numerous choices daily. Practice implementing these skills on your job, at home, or in community activities. Become active in professional nursing organizations and take on leadership roles. Learn how to give assignments to others, taking care to provide the time and resources necessary to help them successfully complete the tasks at hand.

Do you have the initiative and willingness to take on responsibility? In the current downsizing trend in health care, managers must be able to operate independently and make significant contributions to productivity and the financial bottom line. Make it a habit to asking for more work and expand the scope of your current job. Contribute new ideas to management for ways to improve your department or unit.

Do you have strong communication skills? The ability to listen, explain clearly, and give precise directions is crucial. Oral and written skills are paramount in management success, but communicating effectively also means using technology to transmit information. Practice speaking at and facilitating meetings. Volunteer to serve on department committees and be an active participant. Improve written skills by writing reports or correspondence.

Are you a good listener? Listening is a critical part of communication. Employers want managers who ask for and listen to ideas and suggestions. Pay close attention as colleagues state their requests or outline a problem.

Be conscious of letting a person explain while you take in what is being said. Do not interrupt. Managers, however hurried or pressured they may be, need to allow others to express themselves completely. Once you have heard everything, formulate your response. This way, both employers and those you supervise will view interaction with you in a positive way.

Have you studied other managers? Observe managers you respect and those you don't respect and analyze their skills. How assertive are they? How do they make decisions? Are they respectful of employees? Do they listen? Do they accept feedback graciously? Do they follow up with employee issues? Emulate their strengths to develop your own style. Learn how to handle problems by watching what managers do well or not so well. Seek advice on how to motivate others and manage workload. People work hardest for and are most loyal to managers who praise and reward good work.

Do you use professional ethics? Managers must display high moral standards. Do you respect all other employees? Are you careful not to offend other staff? Are you sensitive to diversity issues? Are you careful not to use terminology that others might deem offensive? Do you treat all people fairly? In today's managed care environment, it is especially important to show a high level of integrity and avoid actions that could be seen as discriminatory or harassing or that demonstrate a different care standard for patients.

Can you handle deadlines as well as set and meet goals? The higher in an organization you move, the more pressure you will encounter, so you need to develop coping mechanisms that will help you handle challenges without burning out. Good time management skills are essential. When you plan projects, develop a timeline that outlines the tasks. As your workload and the number of staff under you increase, you will need to become extremely organized. You need to create a foundation to deal more effectively with problems as they arise.

As a new manager, you will want to create a few strategies to enhance your chance of success. Here are some strategies to consider using when you are in a new management role.

- Open your office door and be available and visible. Staff are not sure what you are up to if they can't see you.
- Be seen. Just hang out with staff at planned meetings, lunches, and breaks. You can learn more about what is happening on your unit by hanging around the coffee pot than you ever will in a staff meeting. Be honest and deal with staff fears, like downsizing, redesign issues, and

layoffs. Tell the truth and tell it often. Staff may not talk about what they are really worried about, so you need to talk about what you think people are really thinking and feeling. When fears are mentioned and discussed, you can establish a relationship.

- Deal with conflict. Groups of people and team members will invariably experience conflict. Many managers choose to ignore conflict, and hope that it will go away, or use coercion to get staff to change. As many of us have experienced, this doesn't work well in health care.

  To deal with conflict among staff, start by asking those who disagree to paraphrase one another's comments. This may help them learn whether they really understand each other. Work out a compromise. Agree on the underlying source of conflict and then engage in give-and-take to finally agree on a solution. Ask each person to list what the others should do. Exchange lists and select a compromise that all are willing to accept. You may need to convince some team members that they sometimes have to admit they are wrong. Help them save face by convincing them that changing a position may actually show strength. Last, but not least, respect the experts on the team. Give their opinions more weight when the conflict involves their expertise, but don't rule out conflicting opinions. Creative conflict resolution can be positive for everyone involved.

- Share information. Staff need to know what upper management is thinking and planning. If staff are uninformed, they feel as if changes are being "done to" them, instead of feeling they are involved in making the changes. Use newsletters, memos, and meetings to keep staff up-to-date.

- Involve employees. Ask staff for input and ideas on how to downsize or improve services. Reward innovators and follow up on suggestions. One important caveat: Don't ask the question unless you are absolutely committed to listening to and following up on the answer. Staff resent being asked for input when nothing happens after they give it.

- Give it time. It takes time for new managers to learn how to be effective. It takes time for staff to trust and respect new managers. Be patient. You cannot rush this process.

You can evaluate and enhance the leadership skills you already possess, according to clinical psychologist Toni Bernay (Maltais, 1998). Despite some leaders being more experienced or successful than others, none of us is starting from scratch. According to Dr. Bernay, good leaders first know, sense, and understand. In other words, they understand themselves. It is a way to take stock of strengths, weaknesses, motivation, and values.

When evaluating oneself, a few areas to consider include decision-making strategies, self-confidence, interpersonal skills (such as listening, facilitation, conflict management and written communication), adaptability, integrity, commitment, and empathy. Dr. Bernay believes that in assessing your own strengths and weaknesses, you should evaluate where you are presently, not what you were, or what you hope to become. This requires honesty about the raw materials you have to work with.

Another essential skill for leadership is observation. Notice who the leaders are. True leaders are individuals whom people just gravitate to. Using a true leader as a mentor offers valuable insight into your behavior, as well as discussing what works and what doesn't with an expert. Keep in mind that not all mentoring experiences can be positive. I have learned a lot about how not to behave by watching some leaders in health care.

In terms of how leaders actually lead, most successful leaders communicate effectively, empower followers, have a clear vision, see the bigger picture, see potential pitfalls, and have positive self-regard and confidence.

Leaders tend to fail, according to USC professor Morgan McCall, (Maltais, 1998) when success goes to their heads and they are misled into believing they are infallible and need no one else. One way to keep such egos in check is to realize that leaders wouldn't have a role without people to lead. Therefore, a crucial duty is to empower followers by imbuing a sense of significance, competence, and community (Maltais, 1998). Great leaders often inspire their followers to high levels of achievement by showing them how their work contributes to worthwhile ends, according to Warren Bennis (Maltais, 1998). Maintaining open lines of honest communication is a way to create an inclusive environment. "Too many leaders at times are too guarded," says Hal Rosenbluth, "They should share their emotions, but remain even-tempered" (Maltais, 1998).

## JOB SECURITY: IS THERE SUCH A THING IN NURSING?

Hospitals may be downsizing, but the health care industry is experiencing phenomenal growth, earning a place among the top three fastest growing industries in the United States (McLaughlin and McLaughlin, 1998). In addition to this growth, there is a highly competitive business atmosphere that many nurses would expect to find in a boardroom rather than a hospital. The bulk of growth in this industry is expected and projected to continue outside the hospital in areas that include managed care and clinics.

As the nation moves from fee-for-service providers to managed care providers, there will be rapid growth. HMOs, PPOs, and preventative health care clinics will see dramatic increases in membership and care needs. A steadily rising population of the elderly adds to the needs of long-term care facilities and home health care.

More than three million jobs will be added to the health care industry between 1994 and 2005, with only 165,000 predicted to be managerial- and executive-level positions. The rest of the jobs are expected to be care-based positions, especially registered nurses in expanded and advanced practice roles. Having transferable skills makes nurses more marketable and attractive in these new roles. In spite of massive change in the health care industry, there has never been more job security than as we approach the millennium!

## DISCUSSION QUESTIONS

1.  Why is emotional intelligence important for nurses?
2.  Do nurses in your geographic area use emotional intelligence at work? Why or why not?
3.  How many of Weisinger's emotional intelligence criteria apply to you?
4.  Would nursing practice change if emotional intelligence was required or taught in nursing school? Why or why not?
5.  Are nurses self-empowered? Why or why not?
6.  List ways that nurses can exhibit self-empowerment.
7.  Create a self-assessment to determine your personal empowerment.
8.  Is it important for nurses to be self-empowered? Why or why not?
9.  Is networking important for nurses? Why or why not?
10. Are nurses skilled at networking in your geographic area? Why or why not?

---

**BIBLIOGRAPHY**

Adizes, S. 1993. *Mastering Change*. Pacific Palisades, California: Adizes Institute Publications.

American Association of Ambulatory Care Nurses. 1996. *Standards for Ambulatory Care Nursing*. Aliso Viejo, California: AACN.

American Association of Colleges of Nursing. 1995. *Essentials of Masters Education for Advanced Practice Nursing*. Unpublished.

American Association of Colleges of Nursing, American Organization of Nurse Executives, and National Organization for Associate Degree Nursing. 1995. *A Model for Differentiated Nursing Practice*. Washington, D.C.: AACN.

American Association of Critical-Care Nurses. 1996. "Decision Grid for Delegation." Staffing Tool Kit. Aliso Viejo, California: AACN Publishing.

———. 1997. *Career Development Services*. Brochure. Aliso Viejo, California: AACN Publishing.

American Nurses' Association. 1993. *Nursing's Agenda for Health Care Reform*. Washington, D.C.: ANA Publishing.

———. 1996a. *Registered Professional Nurses and Unlicensed Assistive Personnel*. 2nd ed. Washington, D.C.: ANA Publishing.

———. 1996b. *Scope and Standards of Advanced Practice Registered Nursing*. Washington, D.C.: ANA Publishing.

American Organization of Nurse Executives. 1996. *Talking Points on Hospital Redesign*. Washington, D.C.: American Organization of Nurse Executives.

Austin, N. 1995. "The Skill Every Manager Must Master." *Working Woman*, May, 29–30.

Badger, J. 1995. "Tips for Managing Stress on the Job." *American Journal of Nursing*, September, 31–33.

Beakley, P. 1998. "Are You Smart Enough for Your Job?" *University of Phoenix* (spring): 14–16.

Bolen, D., and Unland, J. 1994. "Surviving Stress." *Hospitals and Health Networks*, 20 October, 100.

Bridges, W. 1980. *Transitions*. Boston: Addison Wesley Publishing.

———. 1988. *Surviving Corporate Transition*. New York: Doubleday.

Brock, R. 1996. "Head for Business." *Hospitals and Health Networks*, 5 December, 62–66.

Burns, J. 1993. "Caring for the Community." *Modern Healthcare*, 8 November, 30–33.

Butts, J., and Brock, A. 1996. "Optimizing Nursing through Reorganization: Mandates for the New Millennium." *Nursing Connections* 9(4): 49–58.

California Strategic Planning Committee for Nursing. 1996. *Final Report*. Irvine, California: California Strategic Planning Committee for Nursing.

Chriss, L. 1996. "Nurses Learn How to Work with Assistants." *NurseWeek*, 30 September, 1–3.

Collins, H.L. 1989. "How Well Do Nurses Nurture Themselves?" *RN*, May, 39–41.

Conti, R. 1996. "Nurse Case Manager Roles: Implications for Practice." *Nursing Administration Quarterly* 21:1.

Curran, C., ed. 1990. "IDN Core Competencies and Nursing's Role." *Nursing Economics*, December.

Davis, C., ed. 1996. *Nursing Staff in Hospitals and Nursing Homes: Is It Adequate?* National Institute of Medicine. Washington, D.C.: National Academy Press.

Donaho, B., ed. 1996. *Celebrating the Journey: A Final Report on Strengthening Hospital Nursing*. Philadelphia: National Academy Press.

Dracup, K., and Bryan-Brown, C., eds. 1998. "Thinking Outside the Box and Other Resolutions." *American Journal of Critical-Care*, January, 1.

Eck, S. et al. 1996. "Consumerism, Nursing and the Reality of Resources." *Nursing Administration Quarterly* 12(3): 1–11.

Federwisch, A. 1997. "Teammates or Adversaries? Your Attitude Matters." *NurseWeek*, 13 October, 1.

———. 1998. "Attitude Matters." *NurseWeek,* 26 January, 13.

Goleman, D. 1995. *Emotional Intelligence: Why It Can Matter More Than IQ*. New York: Bantam Books.

Gray, B.B. 1994a. "Twenty-First Century Hospital Embodies New Concept." *NurseWeek*, 1 April, 1.

———. 1994b. "Changing Skill Mix Reorders Healthcare Delivery System." *NurseWeek*, 2 December, 14.

———. 1995. "Issues at the Crossroads." Parts 1 and 2. *NurseWeek*, 1 October, 1.

Groves, M. 1996. "Life After Layoffs." *Los Angeles Times*, 25 March, 3.

Hagland, M. 1995. "Incent Me." *Hospitals and Health Networks*, 5 September, 7.

Hammers, M.A. 1994. "Crystal Ball Gazing with Leland Kaiser." *RN Times*, 5 September, 8–10.

Keepnews, D., and Marullo, G. 1996. "Policy Imperatives for Nursing in an Era of Healthcare Restructuring." *Nursing Administration Quarterly* 20(3): 19–31 (spring).

Kennedy, M.M. 1996. "Skills Transfer." *Executive Female*, September/October, 27–31.

Kunen, J. 1996. "The New Hands-Off Nursing." *Time*, 30 September, 55–57.

Linden, A. 1998. "Getting What You Want," *Executive Female*, February, 4–7.

Lumsdon, K. 1995a. "Working Smarter, Not Harder." *Hospitals and Health Networks*, 5 November, 27–31.

———. 1995b. "Faded Glory." *Hospitals and Health Networks*, 5 December, 31–36.

MacStravic, S. 1987. "Managing Demand: The Wrong Paradigm." *Managed Care Quarterly* 5(4): 8–17.

Maltais, M. 1998. "Leadership's Leading Indicators." *Los Angeles Times*, 8 June, 3.

Malone, B. et al. 1996. "A Grim Prognosis for Healthcare." *American Journal of Nursing Survey Results*, November, 40.

Manion, J. 1996. "Understanding the Seven Stages of Change." *RN Magazine*, April, 21.

Manthey, M. 1994. "Issues in Patient Care Delivery." *Journal of Nursing Administration* 24(12): 14–16.

Marks, M. 1994. *From Turmoil to Triumph.* New York: Lexington Press.

Mauer, R. 1996. *Beyond the Wall of Resistance.* Austin, Texas: Bard Books, Inc.

Morrell, J. 1995. "Turn Your Focus Outside In." *Hospitals and Health Networks*, 5 December, 66.

McLaughlin, P., and McLaughlin, P., Jr. 1998. "The Seven Steps to Top Performance." *Executive Female*, April, 6–8.

McManis, G.L. 1993. "Reinventing the System." *Hospitals and Health Networks*, 5 October, 42–48.

McNeese-Smith, D. 1995. "Leadership Behavior and Employee Effectiveness." *Nursing Management* 24(5): 38-39.

Meissner, J. 1986. "Nurses: Are We Eating Our Young?" *Nursing '86,* March, 52-53.

Miller, J. 1995. "Leading Nursing into the Future." *Harvard Nursing Research Institute Newsletter* 4(3): 5–7 (summer).

Miller, M., ed. *Colorado Differentiated Practice Model for Nursing.* Colorado School of Nursing. Unpublished.

Moore, J.D. Jr. 1998. "What Downsizing." *Modern Healthcare*, 19 January, 12.

National Association of Female Executives. 1990. *How to Short-Circuit Stress.* Pamphlet. New York: NAFE. Pamphlet.

———. 1993. Pamphlet. *Guide to a Winning Resume.* New York: NAFE.

Neale, M. 1997. "The Art of the Deal." *Hospitals and Health Networks*, 5 April, 38–39.

O'Rourke, M.W. 1996. "Who Holds the Keys to the Future of Healthcare?" *NurseWeek*, 8 January, 1.

Organization of Nurse Leaders. 1995. "Focus Group Notes." *Nursing Issues*, 29 September.

Perryman, A. 1998. "Sixteen Ways To Succeed in a New Work Place. " *Executive Female*, April, 14.

Pew Health Professions Commission. 1995. "Healthy America: Practitioners for 2005." *Pew Health Professions Report.* Washington, D.C.: Pew Health Professions Commission.

———. 1998. " *Pew Health Professions Report.* Washington, D.C.: Pew Health Professions Commission.

Pinto, C. et al. 1998. "Future Trends." *Modern Healthcare*, 5 January, 27–40.

Rich, P.L. 1995. "Working with Nursing Assistants: Becoming a Team." *Nursing 95*, May, 100–103.

RN Special Advisory Committee. 1990. *Meeting the Immediate and Future Needs for Nursing in California.* Sacramento, California: State of California.

Ryan, R. 1997. *24 Hours to Your Next Job, Raise or Promotion.* New York: John Wiley & Sons.

———. 1998a. "Moving into Management." *Executive Female*, February, 8.

———. 1998b. "Super Effective Interview Tactics." *Executive Female*, February, 6.

Sherer, J. 1995. "Tapping into Teams." *Hospitals and Health Networks*, 5 July, 32–35.

Shindul-Rothschild, J. et al. 1997. "Ten Keys to Quality Care." *American Journal of Nursing* 97(11): 35–43.

Shubert, D. 1996. "Hospitals Decrease Nurses' Role: Reassign Tasks to Aides." *Los Angeles Times*, 14 July.

Smith, L. 1993. "Never Fail To Be Gracious." *Executive Female*, September/October, 7–10.

Sokolosky, V. 1996. "Mastering Career Change." *Spirit* (Southwest Airlines), August, 132–133.

Stern, C. 1994. "Communication Strategies." Lecture handouts, September 1996, Los Angeles.

Stern, C. et al. 1991. *Kaiser Foundation Hospitals Graduate Nurse Handbook of Job Searching Techniques*. 4th ed. Oakland, California: Kaiser Permanente Hospitals.

Strasen, L. 1987. *Business Skills for Nurses*. New York: Lippincott.

Sund, J. et al. 1998. "Case Management in an Integrated Delivery System." *Nursing Management*, January, 24–32.

Thomas, D. 1994. "Five Ways to Run Your Career Like a Business." *Executive Female*, November/December, 37–40.

Turner, S.O. 1995a. "Marketing Yourself in the 'Nineties." *American Journal of Nursing*, January, 20–23.

———. 1995b. "Stand Out or Lose Out." *Nursing 95*, January, 13–18.

———. 1995c. "Laid Off: Now What?" *Nursing 95*, May, 94–95.

———. 1995d. " Managing Your Transition: Strategies for the Future." *Surgical Services Management*, May, 40–42.

———. 1995e. "Reality Check: It's Time for Nursing to Face the Future." *Hospitals and Health Networks*, 20 August, 20–22.

———. 1995f. "Nurses: Are They the Key to Successful Capitation?" *Capitation and Medical Practice*, December, 1–2.

———. 1996. "Capitation: Are You Ready for It?" *Surgical Services Management*, February, 43–45.

Van, S. 1994. "A New Attitude." *RN Times*, November, 12–13.

Vitale, S. 1995. "Reinventing Your Career." *Executive Female*, September/October, 43–56.

Weisinger, H. 1998. *Emotional Intelligence at Work*. San Francisco: Jossey-Bass.

# CHAPTER 18

# Managed Care Business Skills

It is extremely important for nurses to have a basic understanding of business methodology as it relates to health care facilities and hospitals. Being informed about business concepts not only gives nurses a better understanding of facilities' choices, but also expands and sharpens their minds. Accounting and financial considerations drive much of facilities' reimbursement practices. Nurses need to be familiar with those concepts.

## ACCOUNTING BASICS FOR NURSES

Cost accounting is an accounting method used by hospitals. It is defined as a method of accounting for total costs of a business, then tracking and allocating those costs to the specific product or service produced. Usually, the cost of producing one unit of service is calculated and then used to determine pricing. When diagnosis-related groups (DRGs) were first implemented in the mid-1980s, hospitals began to determine specific costs per service with the idea of enhancing revenues. Now hospitals must identify the total cost of care for a patient for a day, the average cost of treatment of a specific disease, or the average cost of a surgical procedure. This helps hospitals negotiate capitated contract rates that will still allow them to maintain a small profit margin. Historical cost-accounting data can be used to determine future cost per unit of service goals. Hospitals can then establish performance standards or productivity standards to measure how a department is managing its resources on an ongoing basis.

Fixed costs are costs that are experienced by the hospital regardless of fluctuations in volume of visits or patient days. Fixed costs remain the same no matter how many patients are in the hospital. Examples of fixed costs would be the salaries of a supervising nurse or of the minimum number of nurses staffing a given unit, or employee benefit costs.

Variable costs are costs that are a function of volume or patient days. Variable costs are over and above the fixed costs of operating a facility. An example of a variable cost would be medical supplies for a specific patient, food costs, or the salary of extra nurses above the minimum staff on a nursing floor.

Total costs of care are the sum of fixed and variable costs. A hospital needs to know its total costs of care in order to determine its ability to discount rates for contracting and to set prices for payers that still allow a profit margin sufficient to cover bills and wages.

The cost per unit of service (unit cost) is the cost of producing a single product or unit of service. The unit of service for inpatient care is the patient day. Other units of service include procedures, visits, recoveries, deliveries, operating minutes, meals, and work orders. Direct costing attributes all costs incurred directly by a specific cost center or department. This means that both costs and revenues from a specific department are "billed" to that department. Direct costing compares a department's actual outflows or direct costs with its inflows or revenue from patient care services it delivers.

Full costing includes the direct departmental costs as well as the indirect costs that are transferred from non-revenue-generating areas to that department. The strength of this method is that it takes total hospital costs into account. The weakness is that some costs incurred by a department are irrelevant to the actual revenue produced by the department.

Direct costs are costs that are directly connected to providing patient care services. Nurse salaries and medical supplies are direct costs. Indirect costs are necessary but not directly related to the delivery of patient care. The salary of the director of nursing, costs of engineering services, and billing department expenses are indirect costs. Indirect costs are usually transferred or allocated to departments based on the departments' actual utilization of the service. For example, costs of bed linen are transferred to specific units in proportion to the actual amount of linen the units use. There are many rules and ways to allocate costs to individual departments.

Productivity measures are another method to determine costs for hospital services. Productivity is defined as a measure of how efficiently labor resources are utilized in producing a good or service. In nursing, productivity is defined as a measure of the efficiency of human resources utilized in the delivery of patient care. Productivity is a key strategy to strengthen the competitive position of a hospital. Productivity conserves resources and helps counteract inflation effects, growth, and increased demand for service.

In nursing, productivity is measured by the standard of hours per patient day (HPPD). Productivity compares actual staffing hours with staffing hours required by the patient acuity classification system and is tied into the budget. Productivity measures for nursing in hospitals directly affect nurse staffing mix and staffing ratios.

Budgeting is another tool used by hospitals to document and understand the costs of providing care and services to patients. Budgeting is defined as an annual statement or process of identifying probable revenues and expenditures for the organization. It is an educated guess at the volume of service that will be delivered the next year, and the expenses encountered to deliver that service.

Budgets should be tied to a facility's strategic plan. It operationalizes three management functions: planning, ongoing activities, and spending control. A strategic plan is a document that identifies the goals the organization wants to accomplish in the next three to five years. Most hospitals also complete an annual operations plan, determining what they want to achieve in that year. The budget is the method by which the organization can accomplish those goals financially.

There are different budgeting methods. Hospitals can choose the budgeting method that works best for their types of services and is approved by their board of directors. Managers who complete portions of the budget need to understand the specific budgeting process used in their facility. Nurses need to understand general budgeting concepts, even if they are not responsible for developing or maintaining a budget.

- Flat percentage increase is the simplest method. It develops a budget by annualizing the current year-to-date expenses and multiplying those figures by the inflation rate.

- Management by objective is the process of supporting programs and services and including them in the budget if they assist the organization to reach its predetermined goals. It usually requires cost benefit analysis of specific programs and services.
- The zero-based budgeting method requires analysis of alternative programs and services on three different levels: the minimum level, the current level, and the improvement level. It requires ranking of both new and existing programs by priorities.

Budgets are usually determined by beginning with the unit of service and projecting for the upcoming year, based on what has occurred in the past and what adjustments are expected in the future. Revenues for the department can then be calculated by multiplying the expected units of service by the cost of each unit of service. For example, an inpatient unit could calculate revenues by determining the number of patients expected multiplied by the daily room rate.

Revenues are the monies hospitals generate from providing services and receiving payer reimbursements and contracting offset revenues. Expenses for providing the service can then be calculated by adding together costs of supplies, salaries, benefits, and overhead. Salaries and benefits account for 75 to 80 percent of expenses in a hospital. Expenses are then subtracted from revenue to determine projected profit. When profit is too small, management returns to the budget to reduce expenses. Usually the first place they look for expense reduction is staffing.

Position control is the list of approved labor positions for a department, usually displayed by category of personnel (RN or LVN) and the number of full-time equivalents (FTEs). One FTE can be equated to 40 hours of work per week, or 80 hours of work per pay period, or 2,080 hours of work annually. An FTE is a unit of time, not a person or a job. Creative staffing patterns may actually allow the budgeting of full-time workers as partial FTEs. For example, one person working three 12-hour shifts per week is calculated as .9 FTE, and this would be considered a full-time position.

Employee time off is included in calculating FTEs. Therefore, not all 2,080 hours are for worked time; some of it is non-productive time. Nonproductive time is the non-work time that employees are paid for. Holidays, sick days, orientation, educational, and personal time are all nonproductive time.

Nonproductive time is calculated and charged as a departmental expense. Labor and salary costs are both fixed and variable. Fixed labor costs are paid no matter what the activity level on the unit is. Examples of fixed labor costs would be the head nurse salary or the unit secretary salary. Variable labor costs are budgeted positions that vary with census, acuity, or volume of activity. Acuity is the measure of the nursing resources needed to care for a particular patient. Acuity systems enable the nurse manager to categorize patients based on their individual needs for nursing care. Categorizing of patients helps managers schedule the appropriate number and skill levels of workers needed.

## MARKETING BASICS FOR NURSES

Marketing is the link between society's needs and wants, and the responses by the marketplace in terms of goods and services produced. The marketplace is the environment in which actual and potential buyers and sellers exchange resources. There are marketers who specifically track consumer needs and wants, and then create the products to meet them.

The goals of marketing are to maximize the marketplace consumption of a product or service, and to maximize customer satisfaction to create more demand. A market is the set of all actual and potential buyers of a product. Products are goods and services that satisfy needs and desires.

Marketing is affected in several different ways. These components are called variables. The four variables of marketing are:

1. Product: quality, style, options, brand name, size, color, packaging, warranty
2. Place: distribution channels, coverage, inventory
3. Promotion: advertising, sales promotions, publicity
4. Price: list price, discounts, credit terms

The marketing mix is the specific combination of these marketing variables used to influence a market. Some marketing strategies may focus more on price; health care marketing tends to focus on the product: high quality service or a certain product line.

Hospitals sometimes group their services together in product lines. A product line is composed of similar services that are grouped together (cardiovascular, maternal child health). Product line analysis categorizes the services or products that a hospital provides into product lines. Product line management is a management method that groups similar products under one manager.

Health care planning and marketing is a specialty of marketing that focuses on the health care industry. It is entering its third era, according to Paul Keckley (1994). Keckley, CEO of the Keckley Group, states that the first era emerged in the 1960s and 1970s and was characterized by distinctly different approaches among the three major players in health care delivery: hospitals, physician groups, and insurers. In hospitals, the emphasis was on reputation. Certificates of need (permits to build new facilities) and specialists were used as key weapons in the arsenal to build community awareness and reputation. Meanwhile, medical groups maintained a principled approach to marketing, contending that their patients would do the selling. To them, marketing was a "bad" word. In the insurance market, the bigger companies were transitioning from poorly planned target marketing to planned approaches to products designed for certain industries and employer groupings. Employers bore all financial risks.

In the second era of marketing, Keckley believes the three major players maintained independence in their respective marketing activities, though each became more sophisticated (1994). Hospitals became discount-oriented, much like Wal-Mart. This was due to the recognition that major employers were becoming more cost-sensitive to pricing and plans. Medical practices reluctantly embraced marketing by defining it narrowly as practice promotion. They used patient newsletters, Yellow Page advertisements, and publicity through news releases and speaking engagements. Insurers were in a refinement mode. Sales strategies and product offerings were customized to market segments, and managed care plans, such as Kaiser, Harvard Community Health Plan, and others, emerged to compete for enrolled lives. Employers tested self-insurance plans (setting their own funds aside to provide their own insurance coverage) and tried negotiating discounts with payers.

In the 1990s, Keckley believes, two major dynamics have shaped the future for the three major players: the rising costs of health care and the concept of health care reform. Employers, stung by double-digit cost increases through much of the 1980s, became increasingly aggressive in their dealings with providers and insurers. The result of this new approach was the emergence of more than 100 business coalitions and pursuit of direct contracts with providers. One of the most successful coalitions is the Pacific Business Group on Health, located in San Francisco, California.

The politics of health care came to center stage in Bill Clinton's 1992 campaign. The Clinton camp made universal coverage and health care reform household phrases. They tried several proposals for health care reform, many not successful. The marketplace has changed in spite of the slow pace of reform. As in retailing where full-service department and specialty stores give way to "no frills" mega-stores, health care providers are now challenged to put everything under one roof and aggressively sell low-cost, high-quality goods and services.

Key challenges of today's health care marketing executives include the development and execution of health care delivery system network marketing strategies and tactics. This approach focuses on a single system entity rather than particular provider groups, hospitals, practices, or ancillary services.

The process of negotiation with providers who become part of these organized networks will be another challenge. The paradigm shift from independent operations to interdependent systems requires new modeling and strategies. Roles and responsibilities must be redefined, and the creation of a successful system will require proficiency in both the analysis of appropriate partners and the negotiations necessary to bring the partnership to reality (Keckley, 1994).

The assumption of risk by organized systems is a monumental challenge. Until now, cost management has been subordinate to revenue enhancements. Most physicians, hospitals, and insurers believed they would generate sufficient revenue by simply working harder or charging more. Revenue caps were not the rule of thumb, and essentially the greatest amount of risk was still borne by the actual purchasers of care—employers and their employees. Now the risk is borne by industry insiders—physicians, hospitals, and insurance partners—who provide override coverage and administrative support. Capitation is the rule and the discounted fee-for-service method is becoming less popular.

The planning and marketing department of the future will provide a variety of system-wide services essential to its success: market research and analysis to explore new/improved ways of providing services, measurement of user satisfaction and patient compliance, and tracking of community health status. Budgets will reflect growing investment in relationship management with partners. Marketing communications will be targeted to key customer groups. In most markets, three to five systems will compete aggressively. Physicians will continue to be organized as large groups in a variety of structures and models. Primary care services, not hospitals, will be the single most important critical success factor in each system.

## DISCUSSION QUESTIONS

1. Are business skills important for nurses? Why or why not?
2. List the five most important business skills for nurses in your geographic area. Why are they the most important?
3. List and define each business skill discussed in this chapter and give an example of each.
4. Do nurses in your geographic area understand marketing concepts?
5. Is it important for nurses to understand marketing concepts? Why or why not?
6. List the four components of marketing and give an example of each from your geographic area.

**BIBLIOGRAPHY**

American Association of Critical-Care Nurses. 1996. "Decision Grid for Delegation." Staffing Tool Kit. Aliso Viejo, California: AACN Publishing.

———. 1997. *Career Development Services.* Brochure. Aliso Viejo, California: AACN Publishing.

American Nurses' Association. 1996. *Registered Professional Nurses and Unlicensed Assistive Personnel.* 2nd ed. Washington, D.C.: ANA Publishing.

Austin, N. 1995. "The Skill Every Manager Must Master." *Working Woman,* May, 29–30.

Badger, J. 1995. "Tips for Managing Stress on the Job." *American Journal of Nursing,* September, 31–33.

Beakley, P. 1998. "Are You Smart Enough for Your Job?" *University of Phoenix* (spring): 14–16.

Bolen, D., and Unland, J. 1994. "Surviving Stress." *Hospitals and Health Networks,* 20 October, 100.

Brock, R. 1996. "Head for Business." *Hospitals and Health Networks,* 5 December, 62–66.

Davis, C., ed. 1996. *Nursing Staff in Hospitals and Nursing Homes: Is It Adequate?* National Institute of Medicine. Washington, D.C.: National Academy Press.

Eck, S. et al. 1996. "Consumerism, Nursing and the Reality of Resources." *Nursing Administration Quarterly* 12(3): 1–11.

Gray, B.B. 1994. "Twenty-First Century Hospital Embodies New Concept." *NurseWeek,* 1 April, 1.

Keckley, P. 1994. "Marketing Healthcare," *The Keckley Report* (spring/summer), 1.

Kennedy, M.M. 1996. "Skills Transfer." *Executive Female,* September/October, 27–31.

Linden, A. 1998. "Getting What You Want," *Executive Female,* February, 4–7.

McLaughlin, P., and McLaughlin, P., Jr. 1998. "The Seven Steps to Top Performance." *Executive Female*, April, 6–8.

McNeese-Smith, D. 1995. "Leadership Behavior and Employee Effectiveness." *Nursing Management* 24(5): 38–39.

Meissner, J. 1986. "Nurses: Are We Eating Our Young?" *Nursing '86,* March, 52–53.

Miller, J. 1995. "Leading Nursing into the Future." *Harvard Nursing Research Institute Newsletter* 4(3): 5–7 (summer).

National Association of Female Executives. 1990. *How to Short-Circuit Stress.* Pamphlet. New York: NAFE.

Neale, M. 1997. "The Art of the Deal." *Hospitals and Health Networks*, 5 April, 38–39.

Perryman, A. 1998. "Sixteen Ways To Succeed in a New Work Place. " *Executive Female*, April, 14.

Rich, P.L. 1995. "Working with Nursing Assistants: Becoming a Team." *Nursing 95*, May, 100–103.

Ryan, R. 1998a. "Moving into Management." *Executive Female*, February, 8.

———. 1998b. "Super Effective Interview Tactics." *Executive Female*, February, 6.

Smith, L. 1993. "Never Fail To Be Gracious." *Executive Female*, September/October, 7–10.

Sokolosky, V. 1996. "Mastering Career Change." *Spirit* (Southwest Airlines), August, 132–133.

Stern, C. 1994. "Communication Strategies." Lecture handouts, September 1996, Los Angeles.

Stern, C. et al. 1991. *Kaiser Foundation Hospitals Graduate Nurse Handbook of Job Searching Techniques.* 4th ed. Oakland, California: Kaiser Permanente Hospitals.

Strasen, L. 1987. *Business Skills for Nurses.* New York: Lippincott.

Thomas, D. 1994. "Five Ways to Run Your Career Like a Business." *Executive Female*, November/December, 37–40.

Van, S. 1994. "A New Attitude." *RN Times*, November, 12–13.

Vitale, S. 1995. "Reinventing Your Career." *Executive Female*, September/October, 43–56.

# CHAPTER 19

# Nurses as Political Health Care Activists

One of the key strategies nurses can use to have impact in the managed care industry is political activism. Both legislative and regulatory methods have been utilized by state and local governments to exert controls on the managed care industry and on the ways health care is provided to consumers. In the past, nurses may have considered political activism a skill that was foreign to the nursing role, and maybe even counterproductive to our efforts as patient advocates.

## THE VALUE OF POLITICAL ACTIVISM

Political activism is no longer something nurses can afford to ignore. Being politically active and informed is crucial for any nurse to function effectively in today's health care environment. Nurses have the knowledge, experience, and motivation to influence health care policy. Now we just need to learn to be comfortable with the behaviors and informed about the opportunities that political activism entails.

Several nursing specialty organizations have created resource guides for political activism. Two of the best are the American Association of Critical-Care Nurses (AACN) *Guide to Political Action* (1993) and the Association of California Nurse Leaders (formerly the Organization of Nurse Executives, California [ONE-C]) *Resource Guide to Political Action* (1996). Both of the documents are available for purchase by calling the organizations' offices. Some of the material in this chapter is summarized from these documents.

A healthy population is an important asset to our nation and the backbone of a successful managed health care delivery structure. To protect this national asset, health care and the maintenance of health must be moved to the forefront of society's consciousness. Recently, attempts have been made at state and federal levels to protect the health of our entire population by creating coherent state and national health care policies.

New political forces have been created to influence the direction of these legislative efforts. Many aspects of health care delivery system operations are affected by legislation. In an effort to minimize the negative effects of managed care company policies that are perceived as "bad," recent legislation has been enacted for a variety of issues, including maternal-child health issues, oncology care, and the freedom of patients to choose their health care providers.

Health care facilities possess the resources necessary for the health care community to participate in government, according to the ONE-C *Resource Guide to Political Action* (1996). As care providers, these facilities can be at the core of the political forces actively working to develop viable health care alternatives for all health care consumers.

Nurses offer a unique blend of special skills and expertise that can be used collectively and effectively to express a unified voice to elected officials. Nurses can educate, motivate, and mobilize citizens within communities. The connection between politics and health care delivery continues to strengthen. Pressure will continue to be placed on health care facilities and professionals to provide cost-effective, accessible, and quality health services. These goals now have converged in the political arena with social policy issues, putting health care on the social policy agenda in this country.

Federal, state, and local fiscal crises have required greater government involvement in health care systems to contain spending for public health programs. In addition, the government has stepped in to ensure that fiscal constraints faced by providers do not deny access to care for any persons in need of services. The government will likely become more involved in the future as issues such as agency oversight and quality and effectiveness of care rise in public importance.

From a political perspective, the health care system is increasingly dynamic because of the interaction between government-mandated changes to health care delivery systems and larger economic and demographic changes. As a result of systematic and social forces, more and more interests are competing for limited public resources at both state and federal levels.

Additional social changes are also operating in tandem with governmental forces to affect health care delivery and programs. The number of uninsured and underinsured persons continues to rise, adding more strain on providers in the form of uncompensated care. An aging population, higher labor cost, new and expensive medical technologies, market-based competition, and specific labor shortages also impact the current health care situation.

Nurses must become active participants in the legislative process. Several specialty organizations have strategic plans attesting to the importance of nursing involvement in designing and influencing health care policy. The current legislative environment makes this initiative timely and critical to the future of health care. Grassroots advocacy and support has never been more important. If you are not involved, someone else will plan and control your destiny.

People have power in government because they are the source of information. Access to people is critical to any political action. Access is dependent on developing personal relationships with those in power. The most powerful lobbying occurs when citizens with firsthand information, power, and personal involvement in issues communicate directly with elected and appointed officials. Nurses and other health care professionals can and should play an active role in health care policy formation by engaging in grassroots efforts to educate, inform, and influence public policy makers.

## THE STATE LEGISLATIVE PROCESS*

The legislative process varies somewhat from state to state, but it is important for nurse activists to understand the system by which a bill becomes law. The federal system is similar to the state process and will be explained later in this chapter.

Whether it is federal or state, proposed legislation is heard first in a policy committee that is assigned by the rules committee of the house of origin. Bills with fiscal impact are also heard by the fiscal committees. The committee hearing process is the crucial evaluation or test of a bill before it

---

*Source:* Courtesy of Organization of Nurse Executives, Sacramento, California.

can go to the floor for a vote. Once on the floor, members usually determine how to vote based on the recommendation of party caucuses. Intense lobbying occurs at the committee level, asking members to either support, oppose, or amend a bill.

Bills must be passed by both the Senate and the Assembly before being sent to the governor for action. A bill can be stopped anywhere along the process, which makes defeating legislation much easier than enacting it.

The first step in the process is to generate an idea for legislation. Any organization can determine that it has an issue that needs legislation. An individual can go to a legislator with an issue that may impact the constituents in the legislator's district. A politician who wants to implement his or her own political agenda or identifies a need can do so by initiating legislation. Legislation is often drafted after an issue has received media attention, such as domestic violence or hospital safety.

Once an issue is identified, text must be written for the appropriate code section of that subject. For example, issues that affect hospital licensure would be amended into Section 1250 of the Health and Safety Code. If the legislation is proposed by an individual or an organization, the draft proposal is "shopped" to a legislator willing to author such a bill. The draft is then sent to legislative counsel for review, placed in bill format, and assigned a number.

The bill is introduced, printed, and assigned to a specific policy committee by the Senate or Assembly Rules Committee, depending on the bill's place of origin. A policy committee hearing is held, and supporters and opponents of the bill speak to the issue. A bill has several options at this point. A bill may pass out of a committee with no amendments, may be amended with the concurrence of the author, or may die in the committee. Most lobbying takes place around the time a bill is in the first policy committee hearing. Compromises may be worked out with the opposition prior to the committee hearing in order to keep the bill moving through the process.

Bills must pass certain committees and receive floor votes by predetermined dates in order to stay viable. Once passed in the assigned committees, the bill goes to the floor of the house of origin for a vote. Each bill is debated briefly, then put to a vote. Most bills require a simple majority vote to pass. Bills with urgency clauses or that appropriate money, have taxing power, or are intended to override a governor's veto require a two-thirds majority of each house.

Once passed by the house of origin, the bill then goes through the same procedure in the second house. If the second house passes the bill with new amendments, the bill goes back to the house of origin for review and concurrence. If the amendments are rejected by the house of origin, a reference committee is convened to negotiate a compromise between the two versions.

The bill is then sent to the governor, who must act on any bill that passes the legislature within 12 days after receiving it. However, if it is the end of a biennial session, the governor has 30 days to act. Bills with urgency take effect immediately upon the governor's signature. All other legislation becomes effective on January 1 of the following year.

## THE FEDERAL LEGISLATIVE PROCESS*

The characteristics of the legislative process affect its impact on the American public by the number of bills passed and the prevailing political climate. During congressional sessions, any senator or representative can introduce a legislative proposal to address a need. The proposal may call for changing an existing law or drafting a new one. Many sources draft legislative proposals. Congressional representatives have staff members who usually draft language on a proposal. For very complex issues, the Legislative Counsel's office in either the Senate or the House is called upon to assist in drafting bills.

Executive communications are also a source of legislative proposals. These communications originate from the executive branch (the president's office) and are often responses to a presidential message or federal agency initiative. Once a proposal for legislation is drafted, it can be introduced in one of four ways: as a bill, a joint resolution, a concurrent resolution, or a simple resolution.

An amendment is a rider to a bill. It must be germane to the issue at hand and can provide change to a bill through substituting language, omitting language, or adding language to any part of the bill. The relevance of the language can always be questioned on the legislative floor. If challenged, the proposed amendment requires a two-thirds vote by the legislative body to remain viable.

---

*Source*: Courtesy of Organization of Nurse Executives, Sacramento, California.

The federal process for a bill to become law is similar to the state process. A bill begins when it is introduced by a senator or member of the House. Frequently, a senator and a representative sponsor identical bills in their respective legislative bodies. After being assigned a number, the bill is referred to a specific committee with jurisdiction over the proposed legislation. The bill is then received by a committee, and usually assigned to a specialized subcommittee.

When a subcommittee considers a bill, it can first hold hearings, thus allowing experts to provide testimony on the merits of the bill. Testimony and information compiled by the full committee are published in the committee hearing report. Nurse experts are vital to this testimony portion of the process. Health care policy and social policy issues are areas that registered nurses can speak to and are considered respected experts in.

Following the hearings, the subcommittee holds a "mark-up" session, when amendments are offered that can alter the bill. When the subcommittee has completed these actions, the bill is voted on. If it is approved, it is sent to the full committee for approval. The full committee holds a mark-up session in which additional amendments may be discussed and voted upon. At the conclusion of the session, the committee votes on whether to send the bill to the full House or Senate. If approved, the bill is then sent to the House or Senate for placement on the calendar to be brought before the full House or Senate.

After a committee has considered a bill, it formulates a committee report. The report describes the bill and the committee's reasons for specific provisions in the bill. It is written by the committee staff and approved by the members. The report is used by other legislators and lobbyists to determine the meaning of the legislation. It is also later used by federal agencies to interpret the intent of the bill if the bill later becomes law.

Once placed on the appropriate calendar, the bill goes to the floor of the House or Senate. The Senate and the House have different procedures for scheduling and conducting floor debate and votes. At this point, all members of the House or Senate participate in enacting or defeating the bill. In the Senate, bills can be modified on the floor by amendments, which can change one provision of the bill or the entire text.

If two bills containing similar subject matter but differing in provisions are approved by both the House and the Senate, they go to a conference committee appointed to work out differences in each version. The resulting revised bill is placed in a conference report and is returned to the House and Senate for approval. Amendments to a conference report are not permitted, and members must either reject or approve the bill. The bill is then sent to the president.

The Constitution gives the president 10 days, excluding Sundays, to act on an enrolled bill (a bill already approved by both House of Representatives and Senate) that is delivered to the White House. The president has four options once the bill comes to the office:

* The president can approve the legislation, and the bill becomes law the day it is signed, unless otherwise specified in the act.
* If Congress is in session, the president can approve the legislation by doing nothing. If the president does not sign the bill within 10 days, it becomes law automatically.
* If the congressional session will adjourn before the mandated 10 days have run, the president can fail to sign the bill, raise no objections, and let the bill die.
* If the president does not want the bill to become law and fails to sign it within the 10 day period, he can return it to the chamber of Congress where it originated. This veto may be overridden by a vote of two-thirds of the members of each house. If Congress is successful in overriding the veto, the bill becomes law. Otherwise the bill is dead.

When a bill becomes public law, by the authority of either the president or Congress, the law is given a new number and the text is published by the Government Printing Office.

## YOUR PART IN THE LEGISLATIVE PROCESS

It is important for nurses to be aware of the legislative process and how health care issues affect policy-making decisions. When considering a bill, nurses should analyze it by asking the following questions:

* What problem does the bill address?
* What solution does the bill propose?
* What are the pros? cons?
* What is the legislative history of this bill? Has it been introduced before?
* What is the potential effect of the proposed legislation?
* What is the feasibility of the bill's passage?

- Which special interest groups support the bill and which ones oppose it?
- How credible is the sponsor, and how likely is that person to give active support?
- Do we need to seek the support of any other group or person to enhance our position?
- What position do we recommend? (ONE-C, 1996)

It is important to complete a bill analysis to determine specific conclusions and provide a systematic way to sort out the priorities for action. The process of analyzing a bill can guide nurses' involvement in federal, state, and local legislative issues.

Nurses need to become involved in the political arena in order to influence health policy. What better way to be a patient advocate than to be involved in changing legislation to enhance patient care? Get involved in a grassroots network with a nursing specialty organization. Campaign for a local community health care issue. Become an expert in an area of patient care advocacy and tell your local congressional and state representatives you are available to provide expert testimony at committee hearings. Write letters to your local leaders about health care issues that concern you. Don't wait to be asked to help. Take the initiative and get involved! It will benefit both you and the patients you care for.

## DISCUSSION QUESTIONS

1. Is political activist an appropriate role for nurses? Why or why not?
2. What impact on politics have nurses had in your geographic area? Has this been valued by other nurses? Why or why not?
3. Identify key areas in which nurses can be political activists in your geographic area. Explain your choices.

---

**BIBLIOGRAPHY**

American Association of Critical-Care Nurses. 1993. *Guide to Political Action*. Aliso Viejo, California: AACN Publishing.

Dodd, C. 1997. "Can Meaningful Health Policy Be Developed in a Political System?" *Health Policy and Nursing*. 2nd ed. Boston: Jones and Barlett.

Keepnews, D., and Marullo, G. 1996. "Policy Imperatives for Nursing in an Era of Healthcare Restructuring." *Nursing Administration Quarterly* 20(3): 19–31 (spring).

Organization of Nurse Executives, California. 1996. *Resource Guide to Political Action.* Aliso Viejo, California: AACN Publishing.

# Managed Care Readiness Assessment Tool

**1. Shared Vision/Organizational Culture**
- ☐ shared vision identified?
- ☐ vision shared with staff?
  - ☐ copy available?
  - ☐ staff reaction/response?
- ☐ nursing vision identified?
- ☐ nursing vision shared with staff?
  - ☐ how shared?
  - ☐ copy available?
  - ☐ staff reaction/response?

Board of directors' involvement:
- ☐ documented? ☐ copy?
- ☐ strategy development?
- ☐ vision only?
- ☐ committed? how?_____
- ☐ educated?
- ☐ paradigm shift evident? for whom?_____
- ☐ business development? how? _____
- ☐ marketing?
  - ☐ what? _____
  - ☐ primary markets?

*Source:* Copyright © 1995, Susan Odegaard Turner and Donald Shubert.

    □ population trends?
    □ age groups growing?
    □ age groups declining?
    □ employment make-up?
    □ self-funding level?
    □ payer mix change over past 3 years?
    □ major areas of promotion?
    □ market share by major service line? □ copy?
□ public relations issues?
    □ guest relations/customer service?
    □ focus group?
    □ questionnaires? □ copy?
□ third-party payer liaison? who?_____
□ care/service fragmentation? how?_____
□ intradepartmental communication?
□ interdepartmental communication?
□ hospital-wide communication? using what methods? _____
_____

□ nursing organization
    □ paradigm shift? what units? _____
    □ nurse exec informed? □ in info loop?
    □ vision?
    □ vision shared? how?_____
    □ copy available?
    □ staff response/reaction?
    □ restructuring? how? _____

## 2. Managed Care Strategic Plan
□ hospital strategic plan? copy?
□ managed care strategic plan? □ copy?
□ managed care penetration of market?
    □ trend over past 3 years?
    □ compared to other markets?
    what is ratio between PPO and HMO?_____
_____

    who are major managed care players? _____
_____

□ changes expected?

which hospitals contract with which plans? _____

_____

which physicians contract with which plans (major admitters)?

_____

- ☐ hospital pricing strategies? need to be changed? have MSO?
- ☐ complete provider network info?
- ☐ provider manuals? ☐ copy?
- ☐ managed care reports? ☐ copy?
  - ☐ utilization by major service?
- ☐ payer contract logs, by contract? ☐ copy?

## 3. Educate Stakeholders

| | |
|---|---|
| ☐ Clinical Staff | ☐ fundamentals |
| ☐ Medical Staff | ☐ glossary |
| ☐ Support Staff | ☐ keys/strategies for success |
| ☐ BOD | ☐ transition |

How? _____

## 4. Physician Contracting Entities

- ☐ organization as contracting entity?
- ☐ vision?
- ☐ support? who? _____
- ☐ strategy?
- ☐ cohesiveness?
- ☐ integration with hospital?
- ☐ practice management? who? _____
- ☐ office staff support? what? _____
- ☐ office staff education? what? _____
- ☐ paradigm shift? who? _____
- ☐ opposition?
- ☐ in loop of info from hospital?
  - number of specialists? _____
  - number of primary care? _____
- ☐ physician satisfaction measured? how? _____

_____

- ☐ primary physicians ready to get into contracting?
- ☐ capitation acceptable to PCPs?
- ☐ physician credentialing information packet/application? ☐ copy?

☐ medical staff roster and bylaws? ☐ copy?
☐ hospital-based/contract physicians?
☐ incentives?   ☐ alignment?
organized groups hospital works with? _____
_____
☐ IPAs?
☐ PHOs?

## 5. Capitated Contracts with Risk Sharing
☐ develop capitated rate?
☐ capitated model contract? features? _____
_____
☐ capitated network in place? what? who?_____
_____
☐ subcapitation?
☐ carve-outs?
☐ risk pools?
☐ withholds?
☐ rates not accepted? by whom?_____
☐ know true service costs?
☐ actuarial analysis issues?
☐ financial contract modeling? type? _____
_____
☐ capitation worksheet?
☐ enrollment size determined to support capitating specialties?
☐ stop loss or equivalent?
☐ copies of all risk sharing contracts?
☐ top five managed care contracts?

## 6. Continuum of Care
☐ integrated continuum?
☐ service lines?
☐ matrix management?
☐ service lines not integrated?
☐ missing service lines?
☐ individual departments?
   ☐ Rehab Therapies (PT, OT)
   ☐ Lab

☐ Radiology
☐ Pharmacy
☐ Dietary
☐ Environmental Services
☐ Cardiology
☐ Respiratory
☐ Neurology
☐ Operating room
☐ Outpatient/Ambulatory Surgery
☐ Emergency
☐ Short stay/23-hour unit?
☐ Skilled nursing unit/facility?
☐ Sub-acute unit?
☐ Transition unit?
☐ seamless patient transition?
☐ seamless patient tracking?
☐ contractual arrangement?
☐ community involvement?
☐ alternative care sites? what offsite?_____

_____

☐ department of health services
☐ police department/fire department
☐ building/safety
☐ schools

## 7. Management of Care
☐ local employer issues:
    ☐ major cost containment strategies
    ☐ typical plan designs
    ☐ which administrators are used most often?
    ☐ employers to contact?
    ☐ average premium increase over past few years? _____

_____

    ☐ managed care options used most?
    ☐ major claims costs?
    ☐ potential for direct contracting?
    ☐ if feasible, what should product features include?
☐ staffing model?

☐ acuity system used?
☐ nursing organizational structure? copy?
☐ nursing model of care?
☐ skill mix?
☐ patient focused care? where? how?
☐ culture shock? which staff? _____
☐ transition training? who? _____
☐ managed care education?
☐ community-based model? what? _____
☐ union facility? which? _____
☐ union activity? when did it start? _____
☐ centralized systems, admitting, billing, etc.?
☐ computerized charting?
☐ non-licensed caregivers? what kind? _____

_____
☐ non-licensed education/training?
☐ home health?
☐ health screening?
☐ health promotion?
☐ nursing care vs. ancillary care responsibilities?
☐ cross training staff? what? whom? _____

_____
☐ floating policies?
☐ patient education?
☐ community education?
☐ physician referral/nurse advice?
☐ nursing student program?
☐ new graduate internship?
☐ critical pathways?
☐ continuous quality improvement/quality improvement?
☐ computerized quality outcome measurement system?
☐ clinical standards of care/protocols?

## 8. Utilization Review
☐ preadmission medical necessity assessment?
☐ admission certification?
☐ certification verified?

☐ case management? tools? _____

☐ length of stay?

☐ UR effectiveness?

☐ Medicare days/1,000 patients?

scope of review

    ☐ 100% Medicare

    ☐ 100% HMO

frequency of review: every _____ days

    ☐ recertification?

    ☐ acuity change?

☐ use of criteria: Medicare criteria used? (increases threshold for compliance)

☐ quality assurance interface:

    ☐ nursing QA

    ☐ medical staff QA

☐ initiation of discharge planning:

    ☐ screening criteria?

    ☐ open referrals?

☐ interface between UR and discharge planning:

    ☐ case-specific action?

    ☐ integrated reporting relationships?

☐ UR staffing: usual ratio (wide variance): Standard use is:

    ☐ 1 FTE/60/70 outpatient visits

    ☐ 1 FTE/80 operating beds

## 9. Management of Costs

☐ re-engineering/restructuring

    ☐ in progress? methodology?

    ☐ will implement? methodology?

    ☐ undecided?

☐ mechanisms to manage risk

    ☐ actuarial analysis

    ☐ stop loss

    ☐ UM/QI program

    ☐ monitoring financials? what type of monitoring? _____

_____

    ☐ monitor financial incentives?

- ☐ distribute financial rewards?
- ☐ case mix system:
- ☐ measure volumes
- ☐ capitated amount
- ☐ total costs by procedure/DRG
  costs by payer
- ☐ LOS by payer
- ☐ outpatient
- ☐ _____
- ☐ cost accounting
  - ☐ physicians receive available case mix/cost accounting data?
  - ☐ physicians receive cost/quality data?
  - ☐ capital to support start-ups?
  - ☐ materials cost?
  - ☐ group purchasing?
  - ☐ inventory on site?
  - ☐ capitated purchase arrangements?
  - ☐ standardized supplies?
  - ☐ physician cost/expense input?
  - ☐ pharmaceutical costs?
  - ☐ diagnostic imaging costs?
  - ☐ surgical specialties/technique costs?
  - ☐ incentive for physicians to reduce costs?
  - ☐ utilization of major clinical services for three years?
- ☐ admissions/discharges by physicians and specialty, three-year history
- ☐ patient payer class, three-year history
  - ☐ admissions/discharges
  - ☐ inpatient revenues by payer class
  - ☐ ER visits, clinic visits
  - ☐ outpatient revenues by payer class
- ☐ program/service costs, by service, three-year history
  - ☐ clinical care
  - ☐ ancillary
  - ☐ education
  - ☐ research
  - ☐ administration

## 10. Management of Information
☐ productivity system/reports available to whom?
☐ physician scheduling via office computer?
☐ physician test results by office computer?
☐ database of current experience linking all affiliated providers to track patient through "care episode"?
☐ managed care penetration in local area?
☐ integrated and computerized patient records?
☐ management reports? about what? _____
who to provide? _____

## 11. Management of Changing Environment
☐ updated plan
☐ ongoing education
☐ management of transition
   ☐ awareness
   ☐ assessment
☐ training
☐ recovery plans
   ☐ retraining
   ☐ xreassignment plans
☐ revitalization
   ☐ work task evaluations
   ☐ CQI link
   ☐ link with customer satisfaction?

# Glossary of Nursing and Health Care Terms

**AACN**: American Association of Colleges of Nursing or American Association of Critical-Care Nurses.

**ADN nurse**: An individual who enters into practice prepared with a minimum of a diploma nursing school education or an associate degree in nursing.

**Advanced practice nurse (APN)**: An individual who practices as a Certified Registered Nurse Anesthetist, a Certified Nurse Midwife, a Certified Nurse Practitioner, or a Clinical Nurse Specialist, and who has a master's in nursing or an appropriate certificate as defined by regulation.

**Adverse selection**: A situation in which people with more serious and costly illnesses apply for membership in particular health insurance plans, resulting in those plans having higher medical costs than plans that have healthier members.

**Allowable expenses**: The necessary, customary, and reasonable expenses that an insurer will cover.

**Alternative delivery site**: Any site where health care is provided outside acute care hospitals, such as home care, ambulatory clinics, or freestanding surgery centers.

**Alternative treatment**: Any health care procedure or treatment that is not typically provided in a traditional health care setting nor recognized as "mainstream" health care. Examples include chiropractic care, acupuncture, massage therapy, and Chinese herbal consultation and remedies.

**Alternative treatment plan**: Provision in a managed care contract for treatment outside a hospital. Treatments most often covered are chiropractic and acupuncture care.

**Ambulatory care**: Medical care provided on an outpatient, non-hospital basis.

**ANA**: American Nurses' Association

**AONE**: American Organization of Nurse Executives

**Average length of stay**: Measure used by hospitals to determine the average number of days patients spend in their facilities. A managed care company will often assign a length of stay to patients when they are admitted to a hospital and will monitor patients' care to see that they don't exceed that limit.

**Bargaining unit**: A group of workers represented by a collective bargaining organization.

**BSN nurse**: An individual prepared with a minimum of a baccalaureate degree in nursing.

**Capitation**: Prepaid reimbursement strategy that pays providers a preset, fixed fee to provide all covered health services (for example, $100 per patient per year for a geographic group regardless of what health care is provided or the actual costs of providing it).

**Care management**: Aggressive involvement in management of patient care throughout the care continuum, including case management, utilization review, and ongoing care and outcome evaluation.

**Case management**: A managed care technique in which a patient with a serious medical condition is assigned an individual who arranges for cost-effective treatment, often outside a hospital. Many case managers are registered nurses.

**Client**: A recipient of nursing care or services. Also referred to as a patient.

**Co-insurance or co-payment**: An amount a health insurance policy requires the insured to pay for medical and hospital service, usually after payment of a deductible.

**Colleagues in Caring**: Regional nursing collaborative efforts throughout the United States funded by the Robert Wood Johnson Foundation.

**Collective bargaining**: Professional organization that engages in the process of negotiating contracts between employers and workers in specific bargaining units.

**Community**: A geographic population of people who have required or will require nursing care or services.

**Community rating**: A method, based on geographic area, of calculating health insurance premiums for which employer groups and individuals pay the same rates.

**Competencies**: Skill sets attributed to an individual based on education and/or expertise.

**Concurrent review**: A managed care technique in which a representative of a managed care firm continuously reviews the charts of hospitalized patients to determine if the length of stay and the course of treatment are appropriate.

**Consolidated Omnibus Budget Reconciliation Act (COBRA)**: Federal law that requires employers with more than 20 employees to extend group health insurance coverage for at least 18 months after employees leave their jobs. Employees must pay over 100 percent of the premium cost.

**Consumer**: Any individual who has the potential to need or receive nursing care or services.

**Continuum of care**: Entire health care process used by health care consumer including all types of health care service. Hospitals are now only a piece of the care system, not sole providers of services.

**Cost containment**: An attempt to reduce the higher-than-necessary costs surrounding the allocation and consumption of health care services. These costs may arise from inappropriately used or duplication of services or care that can be provided in less costly settings without harming the patient.

**Cost shifting**: A strategy occurring in the United States health care system in which providers who are partially reimbursed for their costs subsequently raise their prices to other payers in an effort to recoup the unreimbursed portions or limit the discounts. Low reimbursement rates from government health care programs often cause providers to raise prices for medical care to private insurance payers and patients.

**CSPCN**: California Strategic Planning Committee for Nursing, established in 1991.

**Culture shock**: The myriad of emotions an individual feels when job expectations and role functions in an organization change dramatically due to restructuring or reengineering.

**Deductible**: An amount of covered expenses that must be paid by the insured before the insurance company begins to pay benefits.

**Diagnosis-related groups (DRGs)**: A method of classifying similar and related patient diagnoses to provide predetermined payment structures within a prospective payment system. Also a method of reimbursing providers based on the medical diagnosis for each patient. Hospitals receive a set amount determined in advance, based on the length of time patients with a given diagnosis are likely to stay in the hospital. Also called a prospective payment system.

**Differentiated nursing practice**: A method of determining nursing roles based on competency, education, and experience.

**Downsizing**: Elimination of employees and reassignment of functions during a restructuring/reengineering process, usually through layoff, attrition, and early retirement. System analysis may result in streamlining and/or elimination of duplicative functions.

**EII**: The Education and Industry Interface Work Group of the CSPCN.

**Employee Retirement Income Security Act (ERISA)**: Federal law that establishes uniform standards for employer-sponsored benefit plans. Because of court decisions, the law effectively prohibits states from experimenting with alternative health-financing arrangements without waivers from Congress.

**Exclusions**: Medical conditions for which the insurer will provide no benefits, as specified in a medical insurance policy.

**Exclusive provider organization**: A health care payment and delivery arrangement in which members must obtain all their care from doctors and hospitals within an established network. If members go outside the network, no benefits are payable by the insurance company.

**Experience rating**: A method of calculating health insurance premiums for a group based entirely or partly on the risks the group presents. An employer whose employees are unhealthy will pay higher rates than another whose employees are healthier.

**Fee for service**: A method doctors use to charge for their services, setting their own fees for each service or procedure they perform.

**Fee schedule**: Maximum dollar amounts that are payable to health care providers. Medicare has a fee schedule for doctors who treat beneficiaries. Insurance companies have fee schedules that determine what they will pay under the policies.

**First dollar coverage**: A health insurance policy with no required deductible.

**Float; floating**: Requiring nursing staff to work in units other than the unit they are assigned to, based on staffing needs and patient acuity levels.

**FTE**: Full-Time Equivalent. A budgeting strategy used to identify hours for each full-time employee equivalent. For example, one FTE can be one full-time 8-hour employee or two part-time employees. A 12-hour employee is equal to 1.2 FTEs for budgeting purposes.

**Fundamental aspects of nursing practice**: The three fundamental aspects of nursing practice are: care of the sick in and across all environments, health promotion, and population-based care.

**Gatekeeper**: A health care provider who initially screens patients and determines what care and specialists are appropriate or handles care him or herself. Usually a physician, but may be an advanced practice nurse.

**Gatekeeper PPO**: A health care payment and delivery system consisting of networks of doctors and hospitals. Members must choose a primary care physician and use doctors in the network, or face higher out-of-pocket costs.

**Health care delivery system**: An interdependent and integrated set of health services designed to meet the health care needs of a defined community and its residents.

**Health care system**: A corporate body that may own or manage health care facilities, physician groups, or health-related subsidiaries as well as non–health related facilities.

**Health insurance purchasing cooperative (HIPC)**: A large group of employers functioning as an insurance broker to purchase health coverage, certify health plans, manage premiums and enrollment, and provide consumers with buying information. Also called health insurance purchasing group, health plan purchasing cooperative, and health insurance purchasing corporation.

**Health maintenance organization (HMO)**: A group that functions as both a payer, providing coverage for members, and a provider, providing care for members (e.g., Kaiser, HealthNet).

**Hospital**: An institution designed to provide acute medical and nursing care as well as high technology–aided procedures and diagnosis.

**Hospital preauthorization**: A managed care technique, usually mandatory, in which the insured obtains permission from a managed care organization before entering the hospital for non-emergent care.

**Hospital surgical policy**: A type of health insurance policy that pays specific benefits for hospital services, including room and board, surgery.

**HPPD**: Hours per patient day

**Independent physician organization (IPO)**: A group of physicians formed for contracting with hospitals and payers; may be multi-specialty or primary care physicians or both. Often composed of physicians in solo practices.

**Independent practice association (IPA)**: A legal entity that holds managed care contracts. An IPA usually contracts with doctors to provide care on a fee-for-service or capitated basis. An IPA's purpose is to help doctors in solo practices obtain managed care contracts.

**Inpatients**: Patients cared for in an acute care hospital.

**Integrated delivery system**: A contractual network of hospitals, physicians, and insurance payers providing care in a geographic area.

**Integrated salary model**: Typical method in which physicians are paid salaries by a hospital or another entity of a health system to provide medical services for primary and specialty care.

**IOM**: Institute of Medicine at National Institutes of Health, Bethesda, Maryland. Has conducted several studies of nursing practice.

**Licensed vocational nurse (LVN)**: An individual who enters into practice prepared with technical and manual skills acquired by means of a course in an accredited school of vocational nursing, and who practices under the direct supervision of a registered nurse.

**Long-term care**: A continuum of maintenance, custodial, and health services to the chronically ill, disabled, or retarded. Usually provided in specialized facilities that are sometimes known as skilled nursing facilities.

**Major medical policy**: A type of health insurance policy that provides benefits for most medical expenses, usually subject to deductibles, co-payments, and a high maximum benefit.

**Managed care**: Managing delivery of patient care in a way that produces cost-effective clinical outcomes. It is also a term that applies to the integration of health care delivery and financing. It includes arrangements with providers to supply health care services to members, criteria for the selection of health care providers, significant financial incentives for members to use providers in the plan, and formal programs to monitor the amount of care and quality of services.

**Managed care organization (MCO)**: An organization that contracts for or provides managed health care.

**Managed competition**: A method for controlling health care costs by organizing employers, individuals, and other buyers of health care into large cooperatives that will purchase coverage for their members. Insurance companies and managed care organizations will compete to supply coverage for the lowest cost.

**Management services organization (MSO)**: A legal corporate entity created to provide management services to PHOs or IPOs; often created jointly by hospitals with physicians to provide existing hospital services like billing and business office functions to IPOs/IPAs. It is usually a corporation owned by a hospital or a physician hospital joint venture that provides management services to medical group practices. An MSO can also purchase the tangible assets of physician practices, such as equipment or patient accounts, and lease them back to the physicians as part of a full-service management agreement under which the MSO employees all non-physician staff and provides all supplies and administrative systems for a fee.

**Medicaid**: A state-administered program, funded by both state and federal governments for Americans who are uninsured or meet poverty criteria (Medi-Cal in California). This program pays the health care bills for those people, regardless of age, who have insufficient income and assets to pay the cost themselves. Most Medicaid patients are women with dependent children.

**Medicare**: Medical insurance coverage subsidized by the federal government for all Americans over 65 years of age and the chronically disabled regardless of age. This federal program is mandated under the Social Security Act of 1965.

**Medicare HMO**: A type of contract Medicare enters into with HMOs to provide benefits to HMO members. Members receiving benefits under this arrangement must receive all their care from the HMO or Medicare will not reimburse the patients for care.

**Medicare supplement policy**: A type of health insurance policy that provides benefits for services Medicare does not cover. Offered as secondary insurance coverage to Medicare.

**MN/MSN nurse**: An individual who enters into practice with a master's degree in nursing or nursing science.

**National Commission on Nursing Implementation Project (NCNIP)**: Three-year project funded by the Kellogg Foundation in 1984 that dealt with differentiated practice issues.

**NCN**: National Commission on Nursing.

**Network**: A group of hospitals, physicians, other health care providers, insurers, or community agencies working together to delivery an array of services to patients.

**NOADN**: National Organization of Associate Degree Nursing Programs.

**Nursing clinician**: An individual who is trained and licensed to practice nursing according to regulation and scope of practice.

**Nursing discipline**: Applying nursing knowledge to nursing practice.

**Nursing practice**: Nursing practice is built on nursing knowledge, theory, and research. Nursing derives knowledge from a wide array of other fields and disciplines, adapting and applying this knowledge as appropriate to professional practice.

**Nursing role**: Nurses in practice as patients' partners, advocates, and educators; providers of direct and indirect care; and designers, managers, and coordinators of care.

**Nursing shortage**: The perceived shortage of trained registered nurses for specific roles and functions as determined by nursing leadership. Nursing shortages may not be related to numbers of nurses available, but rather numbers of nurses with particular skill sets or competencies.

**Nursing transition**: The process each individual nurse goes through to mentally and emotionally internalize the changes in role, function, scope of practice, and location due to restructuring.

**ONE-C**: Organization of Nurse Executives, California. An organization of nurse leaders throughout the state. Is in the process of changing its name to Association of California Nurse Leaders (ACNL).

**Open enrollment period**: Time during which uninsured employees may join a health care plan or insured employees can switch plans without proving they are healthy.

**Outpatients**: Patients cared for in alternative sites outside an acute care hospital.

**Patient**: A recipient of nursing care or services.

**Payer**: An organization that pays for health care administered to a group; insurance companies and employers are primary payers.

**Physician-hospital organization (PHO)**: A legal entity created between hospitals and physicians for the purpose of contracting together with payers to provide care. The PHO may act as a unified agent in managed care contracting, own a managed care plan, own and operate outpatient clinics or ancillary services, or provide administrative services to physicians. Some PHOs have membership restrictions tied to criteria for meeting cost-effectiveness or quality; these are referred to as closed physician-hospital organizations.

**Point of service**: A term that applies to certain health maintenance organizations and preferred provider organizations. Members in a point-of-service HMO or PPO can go outside the network for care, but their reimbursement will be less than if they had remained inside.

**Preexisting condition**: A physical or mental condition that an insured has prior to the effective date of insurance coverage. Policies may exclude coverage for such conditions for a specified period of time.

**Preferred risks**: People with few, if any, medical problems whom insurance companies like to insure because they present little likelihood of filing claims in the near future.

**Preferred provider organization (PPO)**: A health care payment and delivery system with networks of doctors and hospitals. This system may place looser restrictions on choice of doctors than do HMOs. Members are not always required to choose a primary care physician, and can go outside the network for care, but will receive lower reimbursement.

**Prepaid Health Care Act**: Federal law passed in 1973 that sets standards for federally qualified health maintenance organizations. Among the standards are minimum benefits and formal grievance procedures.

**Primary care**: Basic care including initial diagnosis and treatment, preventive services, maintenance of chronic conditions, and referral to specialist physicians. Primary care physicians are usually internal medicine, family practice, obstetrical-gynecology, and general medicine trained.

**Primary care physicians**: Physicians who provide general medical care (like old-fashioned rural doctors) in family practice, internal medicine, obstetrics-gynecology, and pediatrics.

**Prospective payment systems**: A method of determining payment prior to service, designed to decrease costs and eliminate the broad range of charges from individual health care institutions and providers.

**Quality of care**: The perception of value and caliber of services and care received in relation to cost of that care, by both those receiving the care and those paying for the care.

**Rationing**: The allocation of medical services by price or availability of services.

**Restructuring/reengineering**: A method of redefining and redesigning health care delivery systems and processes with the dual outcomes of increasing the quality of care and decreasing the cost of services. For the purposes of this book, does not include a specified process of restructuring, but simply indicates that hospitals identified that they completed a type of restructuring process.

**Role transition**: The process an individual goes through when fundamental aspects of his/her role functions, tasks, and expectations are altered.

**Second opinion review**: A managed care technique in which a second physician is consulted about diagnosis or course of treatment. Used to attempt to reduce costs; according to some experts, has had questionable effectiveness.

**Shadow pricing**: Tendency of health insurers not to price their services at the same or nearly the same level as indemnity insurance plans.

**Team model**: Staffing method that provides a staffing mix of personnel with different skills, competencies, and licensure who work together to provide care for a specified number of patients.

**Union**: Collective bargaining organization representing workers. Relatively new (within last 10 years) to nursing.

**Unlicensed assistive personnel (UAP)**: An individual who enters into practice prepared with manual skills acquired by means of a course in an accredited school of nursing assistance, or trained by an accredited health care facility to perform tasks and duties under the direct supervision of a registered nurse.

**Usual, customary, and reasonable (UCR)**: Amounts charged by health care providers that are consistent with charges from similar providers for the same or nearly the same services in a predefined area.

**Utilization**: Patterns of usage for a particular medical service, such as hospital care or physician visits.

**Utilization review**: A technique used by hospital and managed care payers in which the length of hospital stays is kept to a minimum and the number of unnecessary hospital admissions is reduced.

**Vice President of Nursing; Vice President of Patient Care Services**: Chief nursing executive within acute care hospital organizational structure. Responsible for all nursing staff and clinical functions within organization. Some may have additional departmental responsibilities as well.

**Waiver**: A provision in a health insurance policy in which specific medical conditions a person already has are excluded from current coverage.

# Index

293

# About the Author

As founder of the consulting firm, Turner Healthcare Associates, Inc., Dr. Turner uses skills she has gleaned from 25 years of experience in the health care field. She began her career as a critical care unit and emergency department registered nurse. She has served in top management roles including chief operating officer, director of nursing, director of education, product line manager, and vice president of business development for various hospitals throughout Southern California. She has provided transition management for organizations during restructuring and on-going organizational and program development for hospitals. Dr. Turner also has worked with home health agencies and long-term care facilities, joining with management teams to redesign programs for both acute and ambulatory care settings. She designed and published the "Transitions in Healthcare" program; a step-by-step guide aimed at assisting health care providers in easing the transition for nurses in the evolving health care industry.

In addition to her nursing background, Dr. Turner holds an MBA and a PhD in Business Management. She is an Assistant Clinical Professor for the UCLA School of Nursing and is a member of the faculty of the University of Phoenix. She is the project associate for the California Strategic Planning Committee for Nursing. Dr. Turner lectures widely on nursing and health care issues. Her published work often appears in national health care journals.